Walk Strong,
Look Up

Books by Chantel Hobbs

Never Say Diet
Never Say Diet Workbook
The One-Day Way
Love Food and Live Well

Walk Strong, Look Up

The Most
Powerful Exercise
for Your
Body and Soul

Chantel Hobbs

Revell

a division of Baker Publishing Group
Grand Rapids, Michigan

Published by Revell
a division of Baker Publishing Group
P.O. Box 6287, Grand Rapids, MI 49516-6287
www.revellbooks.com

Printed in the United States of America

Library of Congress Cataloging-in-Publication Data
Hobbs, Chantel.
    Walk strong, look up : the most powerful exercise for your body and soul / Chantel Hobbs.
        p.   cm.
    Includes bibliographical references.
    ISBN 978-0-8007-2049-0 (pbk.)
    1. Walking. 2. Physical fitness. I. Title.
RA781.65.H63 2011
613.7′176—dc23
                                                                2011014069

To protect the privacy of those who have shared their stories with the author, some details and names have been changed.

11   12   13   14   15   16   17   7   6   5   4   3   2   1

This book is dedicated to those with
Such a Pretty Face.

May you find the thrill of walking with the One
who not only sees your soul, but has the power
to renew your spirit one step at a time.

Contents

Acknowledgments

I am rarely at a loss for words, but when it comes to how I feel about my Savior and the work He has me doing, I'm speechless. Not only do I get to write books about Him for a living, but I am able to help hurting people at the same time. All I can say to Him is this:

Lord, there is no way the girl I once was could ever have come up with the idea I would be the woman I am today. And because I know who You are, and who I'm not, it excites me even more to know the best is yet to come!

To my husband, Keith: When I think of 1 Corinthians 13, I think of you and the way you love me. You truly do bear all things with me, and I know I'm no picnic sometimes—along with my great zeal seems to come great chaos. Not only do I adore you, but I am also keenly aware that the ministry God has for me wouldn't exist without your strength and support. Thank you for knowing when to speak, when to pray, and when just to hug!

To Ashley: Do you really want to go away to college? I've told you we could homeschool you for it. Seriously, I can't believe you will be finishing your senior year in the blink of an eye. You are already making a difference in the lives of many; however, I'm not convinced it needs to be in third world countries! Actually, when I look at the pictures of you cradling the orphans in Uganda, I am humbled to call you my daughter.

To Kayla: You have a unique way of making everyone you encounter feel special, whether through taking a sick friend a special treat or surprising Daddy and me by cleaning the entire house. The world won't always understand why you keep on giving, but you'll know exactly why. We are happiest when we serve someone else, and you get this at a very early age. It's a beautiful thing to watch!

To Jake: I think you are clueless when it comes to exactly how hilarious you are. I catch you watching your sisters and me wage war over clothes sharing or other matters, often due to high levels of hormones clashing at once. You simply shake your head in a way that seems to say, *Wow, all women are insane!* And we are. Insane about you! We love the laughter and humor you provide for us.

To Luke: I'm still trying to figure out how I can tactfully insist your future wife must continue to sing your "Night-Night" song one day—many, many years from now. You are a very sweet boy with a lot of pressure on you as the baby. I get it, even if no one else does. Never forget you are a miracle, in many ways.

To Mother and Dad: I love you both very much, and I am grateful beyond words for the Christian upbringing you've provided for me.

To my mother-in-law, Linda, and my father-in-law, Ken: Thank you for investing in a beautiful cabin in the mountains with a paradise view that served as the perfect place to write much of this book.

To my Aunt Shell: I want you to know how much I appreciate your love and thoughtfulness. While Pepa's passing has been hard, rest assured, he won't be missing any ball games. In fact, he's now seeing them on a gigantic screen and hearing them more clearly than ever before!

To Mary: It's funny how a walk in Cypress Park turned into a beautiful friendship. Each time we are together, I leave feeling as if I have just spent time with one of God's favorites!

To my editor, Lonnie: I hoped several years ago we'd do a book together one day, and here we are. God cracks me up. Thanks so much for believing in my message and for protecting my voice. Be of good cheer! I have no doubt your persistence in getting the hope-filled information in this book "out there" will aid in changing the lives of many.

To Chip: I still wonder if, after the first time we spoke, you imagined I'd have the opportunity to write all these books. God's favor still makes me scratch my head, but I know one thing: You have played a critical part in all of this. Thank you for believing in me.

To the folks at Bluefishactivewear.com: Thanks for making clothes to sweat in that still make me feel cool!

To Grif Blackstone and the entire Blackstone Media staff: Who knew speaking at a Business with Purpose breakfast would turn out to be an enormous answer to my prayers. Thanks for helping me do what I do best, and in case you haven't figured it out yet, "Geek-talk" isn't it!

To my Pastor, Bob Coy: Thank you for your obedience in planting a church in South Florida over twenty-five years ago. Calvary Chapel Fort Lauderdale is more than a home; it has served as a haven of refuge and as a place of great joy, great growth, and great healing for my life.

To the reader: I must acknowledge you, too! First, I am very honored to have your trust as you give me some of your most valuable commodity, time. Know this: I am confident that as you learn how to walk stronger, a new world will open up to you. Thank you for letting me be part of that. All I can say is, wow!

Introduction

It Pays to Advertise

*A*s I waited for my Egg Beaters and whole-grain toast, an old man plopped down in front of me. At first glance, what to my wondering eyes did then appear but a grandpa whom I imagined had a part-time gig as a model—of Santa suits, that is. My first thought was, *Well, the suffering economy wouldn't affect him trying to get a job at the mall for the holidays.* That is, as long as he liked kids, had a jolly attitude, and was talented enough to say "ho-ho-ho" while making his belly jump. But on this day he was sporting ordinary clothes, with the exception of an extraordinary hat. It proclaimed boldly, "Jesus is my boss."

The breakfast joint we were in was very laid-back. In fact, the majority of the main dining area was filled by only one long table with benches. Strangers had no choice but to dine together. As I looked up and smiled to welcome this St. Nick look-alike to the table, I said, "Sir, please tell me about your hat." Without any hesitation, he replied, "Well, all I know is it pays to advertise."

I smiled again. He offered a handshake and said, "My name is Bill."

By the scruffy looks of him and the oil-stained overalls he wore, I assumed this man was not a graduate of the Harvard School of Business or a fancy salesman. Yet the confidence Bill oozed as he said those words, "it pays to advertise," displayed savvy to rival that of any stockbroker on Wall Street. Combine that with the earnest conviction in his eyes, and I can't imagine anyone who wouldn't be willing to buy whatever he was selling.

But the whole point was Bill wasn't trying to sell anything. He didn't need to beg others to buy Jesus. Instead, he wore a hat that basically said "He runs the whole show!" It was a great reminder to me on this day in particular. Just a few hours prior, the curtain had closed on my grandfather's life.

I had received the call that my Pepa passed away just after midnight. For as long as I could remember, he had been there. He never missed a birthday or a holiday. His brilliant blue eyes and beautiful, wavy, silver hair were a hallmark at the Thanksgiving table. I don't think this special day had passed even one year where he didn't well up with tears as he said grace, always making the same humble request, "Good Lord, please keep us true and faithful to Thee."

Just before Bill made his entrance in the restaurant that morning, I had been trying to imagine what I'd say when I spoke at my grandfather's service. I'm not sure if it was the sincerity in the hat-wearing pseudo-Santa's eyes, or the color of his eyes themselves that reminded me of my Pepa. But the fact they shared the name Bill did make me think our meeting and its timing was nothing short of divine.

My grandfather, William Brown, had a quiet and gentle spirit, more so than any man I've ever known. While he didn't use lots of words to describe his faith, it was something I never questioned. His life spoke of God's trust more than any words he could ever say. However, because he was a man of few words, I was having trouble trying to imagine what message more than any other he'd want to leave with us, his loved ones.

In just a matter of minutes after meeting Bill, my questions concerning what I should share were about to be answered. As we waited for our breakfast, I told him of my recent loss. I also let him know I had been wondering all morning about what my grandfather would want said at his funeral.

Bill responded with utter confidence as he looked straight in my eyes, "I'm going to tell you." At this point, I knew I should take notes. Bill went on. "In John 14, Jesus is speaking to Thomas about His death, 'Let not your heart be troubled; you believe in God, believe also in Me. In My Father's house are many mansions; if it were not so, I would have told you. I go to prepare a place for you. And if I go and prepare a place for you, I will come again and receive you to Myself; that where I am, there you may be also. And where I go you know, and the way you know.' Thomas said to Him, 'Lord, we do not know where You are going, and how can we know the way?' Jesus said to him, 'I am the way, the truth, and the life. No one comes to the Father except through Me.' There you have it."

I knew in an instant this was the only message that mattered. And it was a true testimony to my Pepa's character. While my grandfather had many wonderful qualities, his greatest legacy rested in knowing Jesus was his boss too. It went all the way back to him having survived polio as an infant. Then he spent four years of his childhood paralyzed from the disease. He was kicked by a horse as a youngster, and had a terrible scar on his face. Yet he managed to walk strong for his entire life—by looking up! Even after losing my grandmother to pancreatic cancer in the prime of their lives, he never wavered. The substances of my Pepa's years on earth were defined by his acceptance of Christ. His death was an opportunity to celebrate the eternal life he was now experiencing, and to encourage others to accept Jesus as their boss!

As Bill and I finished our eggs, I felt like I had just received a kiss from God. This hand-delivered message was the perfect way for me to sum up my Pepa's desire for everyone he knew. All I could do was cry, finish my meal, and hug Bill goodbye. I wondered if we'd ever meet again.

The service was beautiful. I shared the awesome story of meeting Bill over breakfast, and I read the passage from the book of John. I went on to remind everyone that Pepa was in heaven for only one reason: he believed in Jesus and lived his life with this conviction. I prayed seeds were planted into the hearts of those who did not have such certainty about their eternal home. A few months later, I began writing this book.

With my deadline approaching, I scheduled a conference call with the publisher to discuss the title. The morning of the meeting, I woke up feeling anxious. You see, a few weeks prior, the person in charge of this had sent me an email with a proposed title. I knew it was not the right one. Not because it was bad—it just didn't capture the message of my book. After pouring my heart onto the pages, I needed to be sure the title was motivating, intriguing, and also hope-filled.

I decided to go for a walk down by the beach to clear my head and try to come up with another title to share during the meeting. Five miles later, I had nothing. My mind was blank. I looked at my watch and realized I had ten minutes to get to my car and plug in my cell phone so I'd have enough battery for the call. Just before the parking lot was a little café. I noticed there were just a few folks sitting outside. Suddenly, I had to stop. What to my wondering eyes did then appear? Sitting at a table alone, wearing the hat that read, "Jesus is my boss," was my friend Bill. I had not seen him since the first time we had met, nearly six months prior. I was thrilled to find he remembered me. He asked how my family was handling everything. I told him we were doing well. Then I mentioned I had been working on a book about walking. Just before I said goodbye, I asked him if he had a word for me. Once again, he showed no hesitation. "To walk strong, look up," he said. I was speechless. It was perfect! Bill had no idea he had just titled this book.

This was the perfect way to summarize the only way I have found to truly walk strong: it's by looking up!

Trust me, coming up with a book title all parties agree upon can take months of going back and forth. So the fact everyone on the conference call got a kick out of hearing the story of how I met Bill—and also loved the title suggestion—was a sheer miracle! I knew it said it all.

Walking has become a great passion for me. I have never found any other exercise that has as much power as walking. Walking strengthens my body, renews my mind, and feeds my spirit. While running, going to the gym, using an elliptical machine, or taking a spin class are all things I enjoy, the benefits of each don't begin to compare.

I know this sounds like a lot of hype for something we've all been doing for as long as we can remember, but I'm going to try to prove it to you on these pages. I don't have a clue if you have very much faith in yourself or God at this moment. I know firsthand that trying to tackle a new plan for getting fit can feel daunting. However, if you'll *look up*, heaven wants to help.

If you are desperate for answers—great, they're here. I have seen God show up in my darkest hours, time and time again, and remind me I don't need to look past what's right in front of my face. You are holding this book in your hand for a reason.

In the following pages, I'm going to show you how to walk stronger than ever. I'm talking about how to use walking as the primary source for making deposits into your "wellness bank," which will deliver great dividends. Sure, you'll be feeling better than ever, but your faith is also about to explode as you look up and see God as the greatest workout partner of all time.

From my own story of weight gain, weight loss, and years of diet drama, I have learned that help from above is the only insurance I have. As long as I continue to walk with God, I am confident I can maintain a healthy weight and remain free from my old life of shame and misery. Sadly, many people don't see that God wants to be at the center of everything we do.

I suppose it's because most of the world is too busy looking back or looking around to look *up*. When it comes to self-improvement and meeting the needs of our body, soul, and spirit, society says we should compartmentalize all of our efforts. For your body, join a gym, buy a magazine, or step on a scale—and do whatever it takes until that scale smiles back at you. For your soul, go to dinner with a friend, read a good book, watch a movie, or find a bench to relax on in the park. And for your spirit, pray often and spend the rest of the time wondering why bad things happen to good people.

After taking the world's well-known route to finding balance and contentment with my body, I was always exhausted and felt defeated, even after I began writing books and trying to help others. Walking changed all of this. Walking has taught me the power to simultaneously engage my physical need to expend energy, my soul's need for quiet thought, and my spiritual need to feel connected with God and His creation. I'm certain there is no way I'd still be on the journey of weight loss and wellness if I had not learned the importance of satisfying all three areas of my life on a regular basis.

I hope this excites and intrigues you! On the following pages, I'm going to introduce you to a program I have created, "Walk with Him." Over a period of one month, you'll learn the how, the why, the weight, and the win "walking with Him" works. It humbles me greatly to have this opportunity, but there's one more thing.

I've tried to be careful to present the Walk with Him program in such a way that anyone, from any walk of life, would feel comfortable using it. As with any exercise program, please consult with your physician to be sure you are physically able to participate.

My dear friends, here is my mission for this book: I pray I am able to be a mouthpiece of hope for anyone hurting, tired, frustrated, and feeling worthless who is ready to leave this all behind. With that being said, if this is you, it's time. Let's take a walk, shall we?

Part 1

The Why

1

All I Heard Was
"Get" and "Fat"

wenty years ago, I was a clueless kid entering junior college who had a *teensy* weight problem (I was carrying around over 300 pounds at eighteen!). I'm not entirely sure how I got to be "obese" (such a terrible-sounding word) at an early age. I'm thinking as a toddler I may have watched too much *Sesame Street*. My life's mantra had become, "Me . . . like . . . cookies." There's one thing I can assure anyone who asks about my career path to writing "diet" books: it certainly wasn't the natural choice. Seriously, I would have picked this just after trying a stint as a heart surgeon. And I'm the chick who gets nauseous if I flip past a television show that has a hospital setting.

Yet, here I am, it's three in the morning, and I'm wide awake as I dream about my latest opportunity to write a book about the most powerful exercise on the planet—walking! I won't argue. My education is not conventional. Really, the only "real degree" I have is from the school of "Screw-ups Who Have Been Saved by Grace" (but don't worry, I'm required to take refresher courses all the time). Yet I'm convinced my personal experiences deliver more to share with you than a boatload of degrees ever could.

I don't walk these days because it delivers the "high of running." I say this because after I started training to run marathons, people would constantly ask me about "the runner's high." I'm pretty sure this whole concept is a scam created by the running community to get us to drink their anti-inflammatory-laced beverages. This way we can all support the orthopedic field while we keep trekking along believing there is a euphoric state that exists where pain is relative and enjoyment can be measured in miles. Come on, who are those runners kidding?

I admit, I have spent some time pounding the pavement as a runner, and running is still something I do on occasion. But I'll let you in on a secret: the only thrill I get is after it's over, and I celebrate another survived run. On the other hand, I have found a workout that's anything but new—but renews me every time, in every way—walking! I realize it's a bit old-fashioned, simple-sounding, and straightforward. However, walking has gotten me as "high" as heaven, many times. In fact, I remember the phone call that started my revelation.

It was a late afternoon in the summer of 2008 when Melissa, my publicist, called. She told me she had a request for me to participate in a story for the magazine *First for Women*. They had called her because they were doing an article on walking partners. The editor thought it would be a nice sentiment to include God as a partner—along with a spouse, a child, or even a dog. The editor wanted me to be the "God expert." It's kind of funny when you think about it. What gives me these credentials? I was more than a little hesitant about participating. First of all, I had never really done much extensive walking for my workouts, and off the bat, I thought this might be an issue. Remember, it was an article on walking. Second, I am a marathon runner. This means I take pride in having run 26.2 miles. So for me, the idea of talking about walking as my primary source of exercise was like asking a baby to eat pureed carrots after she had been chomping away on French fries. Yuck! Lastly, while I consider God to be my friend, He had never been my workout buddy. Now, don't hear me wrong. I've done some praying while exercising; however, up until this point, I wouldn't have considered exercise to be time spent "hanging out with God." Also, my prayers were often wedged between songs of loud, fast-paced music. Back then I certainly didn't have sweet songs of worship on my iPod. However, despite all of these reasons, I did tell Melissa I would think about the article.

Within two or three days of the call from Melissa, I began to think about my potential contribution to the article. Strangely, that same week I began experiencing excruciating pain in my left foot whenever I tried to run. I'm talking real pain! Maybe not "pushing out a baby" pain, but pain like "want to rip off your feet" pain. It hurt.

My initial way of handling most things is the same as most other people. I'm a do-it-yourself kind of girl. So this meant that with a special shoe insert from the sporting goods store and 800 milligrams of Ibuprofen, I should be good to go. Wrong! The pain began to get worse after a few more attempts to work out. So I finally gave in and went to see my good friend Dr. Rob Nelson. Dr. Rob was the podiatrist I had run my first marathon with, along with a team for the Leukemia Society. I figured going to see him would help. If anyone knew how desperately I wanted to get on the road again, it was my old running partner.

When I went to see him, he wasn't my buddy at all. Suddenly he switched to "Mr. Hippocratic Oath–taker." He said he had to take X-rays, do an exam, blah, blah, blah! Then, when all that nonsense was done, he had the nerve to tell me my running career was over—for at least a while. In fact, Rob even "robbed" me of my dream to run the Boston Marathon. (I had already accepted I'd wait until I could qualify in the over-75 division.)

I was mad. Not at Rob, but at myself. My "more is more" mentality had stolen something I felt strong doing. So only half-listening, I chatted with my doctor (and dream crusher) about the options I had for continuing to exercise. Rob said two things to me: swim and walk. I heard two things: get and fat. To tell you the truth, I was terrified I'd never find any workout that had the intensity I enjoyed.

As I went home to feel sorry for myself, I began to think about the article on walking. Next, I said a simple prayer. I asked God to give me an exercise plan that would help me stay in shape, keep me out of pain, and make me want to do it all over again. Then I woke up the next morning while it was still dark and I hit the road as a walker, my feet no longer bouncing off the ground.

Within the first five minutes, I was really bored. My body was used to intense exercise. I didn't feel challenged enough to focus. But I kept going, and eventually I powered up my iPod and began to listen to music that had a great beat and an even greater message. Then Kirk Franklin's song "Looking for You" came on, and as I began to pick up my pace and swing my arms, I realized God was there. He was moving right along with me, encouraging me to push harder and move faster. The more I prayed and began to thank the Lord for giving me legs that worked, the more sweat began to drip down my forehead. I'll admit I was a little surprised. Every person I had ever seen walking in my neighborhood looked to be on a Sunday stroll compared to this. I proceeded for the next forty-five minutes to pray, dance, sing, and keep moving. When the workout was over, I looked down at my heart-rate monitor and realized my heart rate had stayed strong the entire time. After I finished up I was exhausted and overjoyed, but most of all, I had recognized the power of walking. That walk, on that day, opened my eyes. Walking was not just a way to take care of my body; it was also a powerful time to hang out with my Creator, doing something He created me to do in the first place.

After spending so much time seriously stressed out about my foot issue, I was now beginning to feel relieved. And after five or six similar workouts, I let Melissa know I was ready for her to schedule the interview with the writer from *First for Women*.

It was near the end of one of my walking workouts the following week that my iPod lost power. I started singing some of my favorite hymns out loud. One of my all-time favorites is one that starts out, "I come to the garden alone, while the dew is still on the roses," and then eventually a beautiful chorus comes in:

> And He walks with me, and He talks with me, and
> He tells me I am His own.
> And the joy we share as we tarry there, none other
> has ever known.

I continued my concert, and with sweat dripping and all, I began to sob uncontrollably. Funny things can happen to your emotions when you exercise. Often, more feelings will rise to the surface. Maybe it's the byproduct of letting stress out, who knows? In fact, back when I was training many people a day, I'd try to predict which client would have an emotional breakdown and need tissues.

Because it always happened, without fail.

However, on this day, during my own workout, it was me. Right on Lakeview Drive, as I was heading back home to get my gang ready for school, I was the one with tears streaming down my face, and I knew why it was happening.

As I belted the words, "And He walks with me, and He talks with me," I had an amazing revelation! The greatest workout partner of all time was available to me, for free, and I had never properly invited Him to hang out until now!

From then on, my workouts were no longer only about me. My heart began to shift from having an entirely self-centered motive (remember the words I heard in the doctor's office, get and fat) to now having the thrill of walking with my Creator and talking with Him about my life, my kids, my husband, my work, and my family. Best of all, I had a block of time devoted to doing something with Him, something He created me to do in the first place! Pretty awesome, huh?

When the writer from *First for Women* called, I'll admit, I was still a little concerned about the possibility of misrepresenting myself as a "walking with God expert" (even though I was pretty sure that three weeks into it I was basically qualified). I'll never forget how this fast-talking, young-sounding, Manhattan-based writer introduced herself to me. "Hi, Chantel. I'm really excited to be talking to you about

God as a walking partner. As you may already know, I am planning to give several examples of walking partners in this article. I will be talking about taking a spouse, a child, a best friend, a neighbor, and of course God, out for a walk." I'm pretty sure God shows up anyway! But then she said something that still makes me smile. "Chantel, we can't seem to figure it out. But whenever we put something of a faith-based nature in our magazine, they fly off the shelf." And I think I responded by saying something cheeky like, "Yeah, that is a hard one to figure."

The interview went really well. I gave her my ten reasons why God is the perfect walking partner. While the young woman took notes and laughed a little, I prayed she would hear more than my humor. I hoped I had properly conveyed how walking with Him could make a radical difference in anyone's life, especially someone who has trouble making time to exercise, doesn't enjoy it, or could use a little more faith. (Did I leave anyone out?)

After a photo shoot a few weeks later, the article hit the checkout stands in every major grocery store. They actually featured my story on the cover. What a thrill it was to have the assurance that, as someone opened up the magazine, they were also hearing of a God who wants to walk with them. Wherever, whenever, we can all show up sweaty and smelly and He'll give us the belief and strength to continue.

Top Ten Reasons Why God Is the Greatest Walking Partner of All Time!

1. He's never late (He created time)
2. He won't slow you down (He's faster than light)
3. He doesn't let the weather affect Him (He makes it)

4. He hears all your problems (and keeps them a secret)
5. He encourages you to keep going (He doesn't get tired)
6. He loves all music (He orchestrated sound)
7. He thinks you're the best (you are His design)
8. He's not competitive (He knows who would win)
9. He'll help you to not become lost (He is a GPS)
10. He'll whisper, "You're my favorite" (you know He never lies)

2

Who He Is

*N*ow, for you to walk with God, you'll need to know who He is. While you may already have a friendship with God, I want to encourage you to begin to think in terms of having an intimate working relationship with Him and letting Him be the boss.

First of all, how can I describe something indescribable? I'll do my best. Unarguably, God is truly the most indescribable Being that a human could ever attempt to contemplate. Not only is He the Creator of all things, He is also the controller. I'm not saying He is the dictator of our lives. We all know we are able to practice free will and make our own choices. However, He has sovereignty. This means every breath we breathe, He gives, and could take away at any time. This sets him apart, big-time!

I get a kick out of having the label of "life coach" attached to my name. People send me thank-you notes, pouring out their hearts, telling me how much I have helped them make some exciting changes in their lives. Trust me, I am honored. But in reality, God is the ultimate life coach. I may play a decent "special teams" coach, but as far as calling the plays goes, He has the final word. Stop and think about what this really means when it comes down to whether or not you enlist Him as your walking partner—and personal trainer and health manager. Wouldn't you have a guaranteed spot in the Super Bowl of healthy living?

But yet we forget this. Each one of us has claimed injury, or quit showing up for practice for a few seasons. And when it came to my personal weight struggles and lack of fitness, I did even worse: I quit the team altogether. Basically, I forfeited the chance to even be on the roster—for nearly a decade. I just sat on the couch and moped, judging everyone else's win/loss record. Silly, right? But have you been there? Are you there right now?

I recently took my kids to a Chris Tomlin concert at an event called "Night of Joy" in Disney World. There, I experienced a memorable encounter with God. As the artist began singing a song he wrote, "Indescribable," I was overwhelmed by emotion. Here I was, holding the hands of my precious children while worshiping the One who bestowed them upon me. The words, "You placed the stars in the sky and You know them by name. You are amazing, God!" streamed throughout this wonderland. It was a small taste of heaven. It really made me think. Why do so many people choose to be frustrated and miserable trying to do life on their own, when what's waiting on the other side is *indescribable*?

C. S. Lewis puts our deficiency in recognizing what we want most like this:

Another reason is that when the real want for heaven is present in us, we do not recognize it. Most people, if they had really learned to look into their own hearts, would know what they do want, and want acutely, is something that cannot be had in this world. There are all sorts of things in this world that offer to give it to you, but they never quite keep their promise.[1]

Doesn't that sound like every claim made by self-help magazines or self-improvement books? How is it that so many people will get so off track in their quest to find love they no longer even recognize it's missing? I believe two words are to blame for this internal war: pride and shame. These are the greatest culprits, always working overtime to steal our daily joy and hinder our personal growth.

You see, to know who God is, I have to know who I'm not. When I take a good look in a mirror, I can see many flaws. How about you? But when I put a mirror behind the cross, and take a good look at it, I can see perfection. His perfect love in sacrificing His only Son to atone for my sin makes me want to be more like Him every day. I'm not saying I'm anywhere close to achieving angel status. (My husband would "Amen" this!) I'm talking about the reflection my heavenly Father sees, and shows me as I look through His lens. His vision is more than perfect. It goes further and deeper than just the physical. Only God is able to see past each flaw and look directly at my heart. Every poor choice, bad attitude, moment of gluttony, and lack of compassion has been burned up in the fire of His unfailing love. He sees me as His precious little girl, utterly dependent on Him for every breath, and I see Him as my Savior.

When I think of this love and its redemptive power, my shame ceases to exist. My need for His grace regularly reminds me who I am without Him, and miraculously, at the same time His mercy and forgiveness give me confidence of who I am because of Him. For those of us who have struggled with a poor body image, low self-esteem, or a lacking sense of self-worth, this is the greatest hope I can describe. When you find out who God truly is, you can begin to accept who He has created you to be.

The very nature of the sin of taking poor care of our bodies lends itself to the feeling of existing in a pit of shame. This convoluted thinking goes with the way it shows up in our lives: on our bodies. Who hasn't heard a preacher say, or read somewhere (perhaps in the Bible), that it's sinful to allow yourself to be in poor physical shape? After all, if Christ lives in us, our bodies are His temple and His home, right? But what troubles me about this theology is not whether it's biblical. Clearly it is. It's that it leaves little room for the power of redemption.

The reality is that every day is a fresh opportunity to take up the cross and follow Him—and trust Him to help you take good care of your body. This means that even though you may be wearing the by-products of bad choices or a lack of discipline, which happen to be displayed by being overweight or in poor shape, it doesn't mean you are living in a state of sinfulness at this moment. Again, even though it may *look* that way—it doesn't mean that's the way it *is*.

The physical state of being overweight has the potential to carry more shame with it than any other sin. In fact, I would venture to say that the depth of it far surpasses what a cheat, liar, alcoholic, or adulterer may experience when they finally wake up, repent, and begin to set out to live a better life. You'd never see one of these people wearing a T-shirt that says "I'm an Ex-Thief" or "Cocaine Rocked My World." Yet someone that has taken poor care of their body will wear their old sin long after they have let it go.

So, if losing weight and walking strong are things you want to do, you'll need to let go of shame. Again, knowing who God is and how He sees you is key, but if you can't learn to lay down your pride after you have repented, shame will be your constant struggle. This is by far the hardest part of the journey to walking with Him each day.

No one is naturally vulnerable, or another word I love: *prideless*. Don't forget, the instant the pair bit into the apple, back in the Garden of Eden, they looked for something to cover up with. Our sin and our mistakes make us want to run and cover up. However, by showing our flaws, we become dependent on Him to take away our shame, help us lay down our pride, and begin to live a life filled with purpose. When we are emotionally naked, our pride is stripped away. However, listen carefully: being vulnerable is not simply letting it all hang out!

In other words, just because you can fit into an itsy, bitsy, teenie weenie, yellow polka-dot bikini doesn't mean you should wear it to your church's beach baptism! Being vulnerable means letting God in, and others whom He has placed in your life, for a specific purpose. You wouldn't tell someone who just got finished robbing a bank and doing jail time what the combination is to the safe hiding in your closet. Also, as you walk with Him more and more, you'll know His character better. This means when you sense He is telling you that shame and pride are getting in your way, you won't be offended.

Very few human beings will let another flawed person tell them they are being prideful. In fact, many marriages have ended simply because of this issue. I often wonder how many generations of one family have been affected due to the pride of a great-great-great-great-grandfather. Our willingness to admit we're at fault has the power to open prisons of pain, suffering, and loneliness. Don't forget: God wants to walk with us to refine us so we look more and more like Him. But if you don't walk with Him regularly, you won't recognize His voice. Too many Christians are living their Christian life out of a suitcase, checking in and out of Hotel Heaven-Bound. Sure, they'll whip out the armor of God and put it on when their own armor begins to stink. But as soon as He comes knocking, calling out "Housekeeping," they bolt! I can remember back in high school when I was working at the local Holiday Inn. Whenever someone would check out of a room, it would immediately become flagged in the computer as "on-change." This term was part of the system that let the front desk employees know the room was dirty, or not available. If we are going to know who God is, we must take our Christian life off the "on-change" status option, and instead offer Him a permanent lease.

Do you know that we love God because He first loved us? I didn't pick Him; He chose me!

Therefore, as you seek to know God, there isn't a need to dabble in lots of different religions or make up one that makes Him more "modern and current." Basically, God's Word needs no revision. And the commandments aren't like the constitution: amending them to fit with the times isn't necessary.

Finally, to know who God is, and to walk with Him, means you will need to claim personal bankruptcy. Knowing you have nothing to offer Him affords Him the opportunity to take you anyway. He loves me. He loves you. He accepts me. He accepts you. We don't need any modifications for Him to choose to pay our debt. It is finished. He knows we're broke and burdened, yet He still offers us a place of rest. He doesn't care if we're fat, wrinkled, diseased, bitter, abused, abusive, wealthy, or homeless. We are His, and He wants to walk with each of us, each and every day.

3

Walking from Accepted to Acceptable

I'm troubled. I've read emails from believers confessing their internal struggle with a lack of desire to be disciplined when it comes to regular exercise and healthy eating. I've actually heard the reason, "I'm too busy serving in my church to work out." This is concerning. At the same time, I've read some notes that sound more like self-loathing than self-acceptance. Statements like, "Everyone's going to have some cross to bear. Guess mine is going to be being fat for the rest of my life." Hmm. This is not good either.

This defeated-sounding soul is walking a dangerous line, implying God makes some people overweight as an opportunity for them to remain humbly serving Him. If this were true, we may also assume He makes a child have cancer so the parents can learn to depend on the kindness of strangers and get good at dealing with their anger issues. Come on! An excerpt from a note I received once:

Chantel, if God loves me no matter what, doesn't He want me to be happy? Exercise just doesn't make me happy!

How I wanted to respond: "You poor thing! Now I'm not happy thinking you're not happy when you hear me always talking about how exercise can make you happier!"

A bit sarcastic, I know. But seriously, here's how I really responded:

My dear friend, God knows you're happiest in the center of His will. It's never going to be His will for you to miss out on the joy that comes from feeling strong and healthy, if you have been given the physical ability to do so.

I hope no one reading this took offense to either reaction. And don't worry, my sympathetic side does come out more often than not! Don't forget, I was the 350-pound girl who walked into a gym, entirely humiliated. Today, I don't write books in hopes of being popular or perhaps starring as a trainer in a weight-loss reality show. Sure, I could write happy books about walking through the tulips with Jesus and smelling every flower along the way while losing weight. But I'd never be addressing reality.

Some folks have accepted that a lack of care or concern for our bodies is sin, while others are haphazardly taking a lackadaisical attitude as they sit back in a pew, chomping away on a candy bar, lacking the energy to fight the enemy who has sold them a bill of goods that says what kind of shape they're in doesn't matter. Yes, sadly, in some circles of Christendom, "being out of shape" can be laughed about, joked about, and skimmed over—with a bucket of fried chicken and some peach cobbler. Meanwhile, the many prayer requests for saints needing healing after a heart attack, stroke, or diabetic-related infection require a prayer chain, or mass email to the whole congregation. Oh, I imagine I've just stepped on some toes. But before you sit down and send me a well-intentioned note or message on Facebook, stop and ask yourself this: What did Christ mean when He said:

I beseech you therefore, brethren, by the mercies of God, that you present your bodies a living sacrifice, holy, acceptable to God, which is your reasonable service. (Rom. 12:1 NKJV)

Was this a suggestion, or a command? And if we can agree that it does sound like much more than a "nice idea," then how do we present ourselves as acceptable if we are willing to accept a life of excuse-making that prohibits this from being possible?

I don't believe our bodies are at the height of holiness when they are bound to regular overindulgences. However, because every human has many God-given appetites and necessities, the process of fulfilling these can open a Pandora's Box to overindulgence. So any nonexercising, regularly overfed person can be just as guilty of not practicing this verse in Romans 12 as a drunk, a person whose mind is controlled by lust, or a chain-smoker. The struggle to be a living sacrifice will be present for each one of us on earth. Just because a person may lose weight and look awesome for a nice "after" photo doesn't insure a holy body forever—or even that one exists in the photo, for that matter. Remember, only God can see our hearts. Be careful not to allow someone else's physical manifestations of your version of a holy life or an acceptable body cause you to feel like a "flop" trying to manage your own.

39

This chapter may be striking a nerve for you. But don't worry; it's doing the same for me. I can run into the grocery store and think I'm just getting a loaf of bread and leave feeling inadequate. There isn't a magazine at the checkout that doesn't try to make each one of us feel like this. Why else would we plunk down five bucks on a whim for something that we'll throw away in no time, unless we thought there was some serious value to it?

You see, friends, I take the liberty of saying these things because I'm guilty too. Remember: we can recognize only things that are familiar. I've been there. I've made the excuses. I've been overbooked, and under-prayed-up. I've done the Facebook status update, "just trying to get it all done." But in reality, how hard am I trying if I have time to go on Facebook?

Here are three things we can do to reap a more holy body and life:

1. **Don't let your schedule, even if it's tied up serving others, cause you to sacrifice being healthy or shut God out.** Sometimes a secret craving for public praise will cause us to blow off quiet worship, where we could be begging for His supernatural strength to end our private battles. I know a woman who was so busy homeschooling, teaching kids' choir, handling the neighborhood newsletter, and visiting a nursing home that she claimed to have time only for fast-food most nights. When I suggested an early morning walk for her to pray and exercise, she laughed. Then she told me this wouldn't be possible. She said she was already getting up at the crack of dawn to do her housework. I had no choice but to keep it real. I told her that some of the stuff she was doing was great—but it was also costing

her greatly. God doesn't want our sacrifices to be at the expense of our health and the joy that comes from having a real friendship with Him.

2. **We need to accept our weaknesses as they are at this moment. However, be careful that you don't use your admission as ammunition to make provision for the flesh.** Here's how this breaks down: if you know that ice cream is your greatest food temptation on the planet, telling yourself ice cream is evil won't help. Especially because some people can open a pint of Ben and Jerry's Cherry Garcia, eat three spoonfuls, and put it back in the freezer. These folks derive God-given pleasure from this stuff! And downing a pint in 15 minutes doesn't make you a loser. It just means you have a weakness for frozen pieces of dark chocolate mixed in with creamy vanilla bean–flavored ice cream laced with large chunks of perfect cherries. So how do you avoid this inevitable struggle? You recognize your opponent and run! Seriously. Until your struggle with overeating ice cream is controllable, inform your family that Ben and Jerry are banned from visiting. Not forever. Because the beauty of smothering a fire comes from seeing the ashes rise up. In other words, there will come a time when a taste of something will be enough. But by learning to handle your weakness better, the internal flame lit inside you, desiring to please God, will stay bright. If you deny your weaknesses, or give in to them, you're essentially adding the fuel of ignorance or of guilt from overindulgence. Both will sabotage your ability to be more holy and serve God sacrificially.

3. **Grow up! The more mature your relationship with God, the more you will seek His approval.** This happens only

with an investment in time spent getting to know the nature of His love. Also, don't be confused by the word I just used, referencing Roman 12 again: *acceptable*. I realize I have already taken the time in the previous chapter to remind you that you're accepted, no matter what. But we're talking about moving past *accepted* and desiring to be *acceptable*. I'll explain more in a moment. But know this: there is an unspeakable joy that comes from serving God and wanting to please Him more and more. However, you may never get there if you can't wrap your brain around His unconditional love first.

I'll never forget learning the difference between accepted and acceptable. The first week after I got married, I wanted to cook my new husband, Keith, the perfect roast, just like his mom had made him for years. Well, I'm sure you can imagine what happened. Whether it was my lack of experience, or that he was missing his mommy, my meal didn't measure up. Here's how he put it at the dinner table: "Sweetheart, let's call my mom and find out how she makes her roast." Huh? I remember saying something like, "You're such an insensitive jerk!" You see, in my mind, all I wanted to do was please him. In his mind, just attempting to make the meal had accomplished that. His comment was more about improving the flavor. Being barely twenty-one and a bit immature, I had trouble seeing this. But now, eighteen years later, I know Keith's heart. I have heard many compliments on my cooking over the years for him. I'd like to think that same conversation wouldn't offend me as much if it were to take place today. Our relationship with God is much the same as this situation. We need to move past the "newlywed phase" of getting to know Him. We should seek to enjoy the depth of a mature and intimate relationship with Him, and to do that, understanding the difference between being accepted and acceptable is key.

The only way to grow up and grow old with Him is by realizing His love for us is already so deep that nothing we could do (lose weight, eat healthier, exercise more, sin less) would make Him think we're more valuable. If we'd grab hold and savor His sweet adoration of us, His children, then doing things to please Him with every area of our lives would be more like acts of worship and gratitude than pathetic attempts to feel more worthy. In reality, there is nothing we could ever do or accomplish to become more acceptable. Therefore, seeking to become more acceptable has nothing to do with trying to earn His acceptance and everything to do with understanding the magnitude of it.

4

Your Race Is Yours

*I*sn't it amazing how much noise exists in our lives? Getting away from it is the main reason I love walking. We give God the podium to speak while we quietly listen.

Now it's time we get to business. Everything I've said up until now has been necessary. If I hadn't taken the time to talk about these things, it would be like sending you into a desert without any food or water. And the desert can be a beautiful place with both—or a place of death without either. I want to help you find true beauty in walking with Him, in every way.

I have discussed how the finish line to ultimate wellness will never be obtained here on earth. However, there is something to be said for entering regular races. Think of these as tests, trials, practice runs—essentially, qualifiers. An Olympic gold medal for swimming isn't available to everyone who has ever stepped into a swimming pool. Anyone I've ever heard interviewed after receiving one has shared how it represented much more than the moment they stood on the podium and the medal was placed around their neck. It represented a willingness to go the distance, no matter what.

This chapter is important because although I hope we are all working toward the same finish line, our practice runs along the way will be very unique. Not everyone needs to lose 50 pounds. Some need to lose 150 pounds, and at the same time, weight may not even be an issue for others. Instead, for some folks, it's all about feeling better and having more energy for living. For them, focusing on the physical benefits of walking is much further off in the distance. Know this now: your race is just that, *yours*! And I have a friend named Cheryl to thank for showing me this.

In past years, I have been a running coach with The Leukemia and Lymphoma Society. This means I have been a part of training folks to complete either a half or full marathon. I have found this to be lots of fun and very rewarding. However, last year I wanted to take my passion for walking and put it to the test. So instead of training a group to run a race, I put together a group of people in my community and trained them to walk a half marathon. This is 13.1 miles. This assembly of folks was wide-ranging. Some were already in great shape and somewhat athletic. Some already exercised two or three times a week and were using this event to kick it up a notch. And then there were many who up until this point thought walking a mile was a medal-worthy feat! Or at least, worth a hot fudge sundae.

Diane fell into this last group. She was one of those people who tested my coaching skills on every level. Within the first few training sessions, I knew we had a problem. Diane kept showing up with a friend named BlackBerry, also known as a cell phone. Throughout most of the workouts she'd stop to regularly update her Facebook status. I'd look over her shoulder and see her typing something like, "I'm feeling tired, my feet are hurting." As I'd catch her doing this I wanted to scream, "Lady, you'll feel better sooner if you get off your phone and move your feet faster so you can get this over with!" But for the most part, I held back each week.

However, as the race day began to close in on us, I knew something would have to give. The rest of the team was going further and getting faster, while the only thing Diane was getting quicker at was her texting skill. I became worried. Up until this point, Diane had never once completed the distance at a training session. Each week I had always needed to turn her around early, or else she was going to make everyone else wait a couple hours. Basically her pace would make a snail look like Jamaican Olympic gold-medalist Usain Bolt on his best day. Okay, I may be over-exaggerating a bit. But Diane was without any sense of urgency whatsoever!

The last training day before the race arrived, I'd had it. At the beginning of the session I told Diane to hand over her BlackBerry. The good news was she finished the whole distance that day. The bad news was she got lost and it took her several hours to find her way back! I knew, at this point, prayer was pretty much all I had to offer her.

I committed to walk the race with a close friend, Cheryl. She had a nagging hip injury and was worried she wouldn't finish. I had to make sure she did. The national anthem was played, the gun went off, and my entire walking team hit the road. I was excited, but also nervous about Cheryl.

It was crowded. Within the first few miles, I lost sight of almost everyone I knew except Cheryl. The first six miles were a breeze. We were feeling strong. It was at that point the race course took us into a park for the next three miles. The neat part about this was how, as we entered, we could wave to those ahead of us who were exiting. So this was a great place for me to see just about everyone on my team and track their progress. It was also my husband Keith's first running race, so I was happy to see him going strong. The only thing that troubled me was I hadn't spotted Diane anywhere.

Cheryl and I eventually finished the miles in the park, and then we approached mile ten. We were getting excited. It wouldn't be long until we were finished. And then, all of a sudden—it wasn't a bird or a plane, and it wasn't Superman I spotted up ahead—it was Diane! I was speechless. So was my race-day partner. Immediately, as we picked up our pace to catch up to her, I began to prepare for the friendly confrontation about to take place. I'd say something like, "Seriously, Diane, you tricky-trickster! You waited until today to unleash the inner-athlete inside. I've been losing sleep worried you wouldn't finish!" But I never got the chance to give this well-rehearsed speech. When we finally caught up to her, Cheryl excitedly (yet with a twinge of a jealous disbelief) proceeded to congratulate her for being so far ahead of us. She even said to Diane, "How did you do it?"

Diane had a very puzzled look on her face, and said, "I really have no idea. I even stopped at a hotel to use the bathroom." I was shocked. Here, I had barely let Cheryl breeze into a porta-a-potty, and I had timed her with a generous thirty-second pee break. *And Diane made it into a lobby, inquired about the restroom's whereabouts, and did her business? Strange*, I thought.

Then I said, "Wow, you must be on a mission today, girl!" To that she responded, "Yes, I am! Especially because I've got some cash now to buy some pancakes with after this is over. I saw my bank's ATM a few miles back, so I stopped to take out some money." *This is insanity!* I decided, and couldn't keep the thought to myself. But right before I barked, Cheryl chimed in. "Diane, you must be moving fast. I can't believe we didn't see you somewhere back at the park."

And the game of Clue was over. Diane simply said, "What park?" I said, "Oh, never mind, it was a ways back."

Everyone on my team finished the race that day. As Diane got her medal, I got much more than that: I got a glimpse of the real race. Sure, there was a small part of me that wanted to scream, "You cheater! You didn't even do the whole thing." But this feeling was entirely swallowed up in the emotion of watching her hug all her friends, and then hearing her say, "I can't believe I actually did it. I've never done anything like this in my entire life!" I felt like I had witnessed someone winning the lottery of life!

While Diane was still taking in the moment, nearby was the actual winner of the race, crying because he didn't finish fast enough to use his time to qualify for another event. And in the distance, a mom was holding her infant daughter in one arm while she smiled for a picture with the rest of her group of cancer-surviving friends she'd finished with. My partner, Cheryl, joyfully hobbled home with a medal in one hand and ice for her throbbing hip in the other. And I had the extreme pleasure of kissing my husband, Keith, because he had just experienced something very special that up until this point he had only heard me describe.

All of us finished the race that day, and celebrated for very different reasons.

Put your race in perspective. What are you really trying to qualify for? Are you so focused on getting to a specific number on the scale that you can't even enjoy the taste of the fresh fruit that's helping you get there?

Or do you feel frustrated because someone is pressuring you to go at their pace, when you know you would do quite well if you could slow down and stay steady? As you set out to utilize the power of walking more in your life, you'll also need to exercise boldness to not allow anyone else's race to define yours. Your race is personal and the finish line is relative. While some may say Diane shouldn't have gotten a medal that day (she did miss almost a third of the actual race), I'd say they are wrong. She didn't knowingly skip those miles. Instead, she stayed on the course she saw ahead of her and then celebrated reaching the finish. No one else dared to take away her race by letting her know what she had missed. It didn't matter. She did exactly what she had set out to do.

Your race is yours!

What would you like to accomplish in the next four weeks?

_____

_____

Is this realistic and relative to you? Why?

_____

_____

In what way would you like to see your faith strengthened?

_____

_____

In what ways does your relationship with food need to improve?

_____

_____

Is improving your fitness a priority?

_____

_____

How are you willing to sacrifice to make this happen?

_____

_____

For the record, there are no wrong answers here. Just be careful to make your goals challenging, or else there would be nothing to celebrate!

5

Don't Be Afraid of the Dark

For with You is the fountain of life;
In Your light we see light.

Psalm 36:9 NKJV

*W*alking with a friend in the dark is better than walking alone in the light." You'd be shocked to know that Helen Keller was the person who said this. A woman who spent her life both deaf and blind, claiming to be an expert walker? And not just when it came to walking in the dark, something she obviously knew well, but also when it came to walking in the light. How could she possibly know anything about light?

Too much light can be a bad thing. Have you ever been driving and someone heading in the opposite direction has their high beams on? You can feel blinded by the light! I

51

think so many people can't see their way out of their pit of despair because they are always looking for light. Many people spend so much time seeking information, to become "enlightened," they are never forced to truly trust anyone or anything. When one thing doesn't work, they just move on, desperately looking for a new ray of hope to be their beacon of light. For someone on a quest to lose weight and improve their fitness, it's often the search for a new book, a new diet, or a famous face who has turned into a quick-weight-loss expert. (At least for as long as their contract is in effect!)

I've met countless people who are beams of information when it comes to the accumulation of knowledge about health or how to lose weight. These folks know lots about calories and carbs, yet they still seem to slam into a wall of hopelessness and misery in these areas on a regular basis.

I remember going with a friend to visit her mother's home. She had asked me to tag along so I could meet and counsel with her mother regarding her weight. Apparently my friend's mom, Theresa, had just been told by a doctor she was at risk for premature death due to her obesity. As I entered Theresa's lovely and meticulous home, I hugged this small-framed, heavy woman. She was about 5′1″ and 275 pounds.

Within just a few minutes, she began to sob. She told me that for at least the past twenty years, she had been at least 100 pounds overweight. Even though she had lost and gained 20 pounds here and there, she had never felt like the battle was getting any easier. As we spoke, she sat behind a desk in her beautifully decorated home office. As she continued to share I found myself fully engaged, but also counting. Not the number of times she said she had tried to lose weight in the past—instead, I counted at least twenty-five "diet" books on the shelves behind her. It totally shocked me. In fact, I'm quite sure she hadn't missed purchasing any that had come out in the past five years, including two of mine! It made me wonder: Why was she still such a mess, with so much information and help on hand? Had she bought these books only so she could pretend to care? No, that was nonsense. I imagine she felt very uncomfortable having them all on display with me sitting there. This would be like a friend showing me their impressive wine collection while begging to go to an AA meeting. It was a humiliating situation for her, I'm quite sure.

Yet, while Theresa had everything she needed to know how to lose weight, and why—from a holistic, spiritual, and even trendy perspective—the truth was clear. Her impressive library of "health and fitness" books (so great in fact the local bookstore manager probably rolled out a red carpet and handed her a latte when she pulled into the parking lot) did nothing for her.

Sure, I believed this woman had taken genuine interest in learning how to lose weight. And this was commendable, but it didn't equate to consistent cardio.

I knew spending time discussing the benefits of exercise and the reasons oatmeal is good for you was going to be a waste of time for both of us. Also, if she had actually read all of those books, she would be much closer to having a nutrition degree than I was. Instead, I wanted to hear something much deeper from her and I needed to offer her an explanation. She couldn't figure out how, with all those books on hand, it was possible for her to be struggling more than ever. So I asked, "Why is it today, more than on the day you threw down good money for all these books, you believe you are really ready to lose weight and get more fit?"

Her answers were raw and unrehearsed. They had nothing to do with aesthetics, such as being able to shop in stores for skinny women, or boldly walk down a beach in a bathing suit. She said, "It's no longer only about me. I'm sick and tired of being an embarrassment to my family." And then with more tears streaming down her face, she said, "And I'm sick of disappointing God, when I love Him so much."

And then I knew exactly why *today* was different for her. I too had experienced that same day, years prior. It was when I finally figured out that all my knowledge, great attempts, and even my solid belief in God had done me no good. All the light I had created was blinding me.

I told Theresa about the beauty I found in the dark. And how not seeing past today was a good thing. I shared how even with an amped-up amount of info, I had never been charged up enough to change. The only way I was able to finally see my way out of this painful prison was by shutting my eyes on a daily basis. I surrendered what I knew for what I needed, and that made all the difference. I needed real and regular hope. So did she. I needed a real, unpretentious friendship. So did she. I needed a hand to hold that was always available, even in the middle of the night when my fears tried to overpower me. So did she.

And I needed someone with the ability to lead me down a road that had seemed to swallow up my pride and make me feel unworthy every time I traveled on it in the past. She needed this desperately. I didn't need to give her a nice "You can do it" speech, because without God, neither she nor I could. Only God was—and is—capable of giving me what I need. And only God could give it to Theresa, too.

As you begin the next month of your life, on a new journey walking with God, don't be afraid to go out in the dark while holding tightly to His hand. It's time to take what you've tried and what you know, and leave it behind. All the light you need for the moment will arrive just in time, as you close your eyes. Trust the Light of the World to take you down the road He's designed for your life. He wants nothing more than to blindfold you from your past, and hide you from fearing the future. I think I've figured out why a woman who was blind, Helen Keller, could claim walking in the dark with a friend was better than walking in light alone. It's because she was forced to have utter faith, to trust someone else to lead her. Will you do the same?

> How exquisite your love, O God!
> How eager we are to run under your wings,
> To eat our fill at the banquet you spread
>   as you fill our tankards with Eden spring water.
> You're a fountain of cascading light,
>   and you open our eyes to light.

Psalm 36:9 Message

If the Shoe Fits . . .

*J*ust before you hit the road, you need to be sure you have the right gear! Just because a shoe fits, wait! Don't buy it just yet. A pair of sneakers is the only piece of equipment you're going to need to get started on your Walk with Him program. Sure, having a fancy stopwatch is great. A pedometer is nice. And a heart-rate monitor is total luxury. But really, I'd rather see you intensely walking down the street in an old bridesmaid's dress with the right shoes on than see you wearing well-matching workout get-up and a pair of old, worn-out, ill-fitting sneakers. Catch my drift?

Know this: if you don't invest in the right shoes, there is a good chance you'll eventually be contributing to an orthopedist's or a podiatrist's kids' college fund. There is no way to constantly pound weight on your feet and not be at risk for some injuries. And as I have learned the hard way, if you have carried around excess weight in the past, your body's structure is already compromised. This means you are more prone to have pain and problems because of the damage done to your body due to the stress of excess weight. If you are clueless so far when it comes to having foot pain, that is great. But still plan on using this chapter to be sure you never find out what it's like!

There are facts you need to know about the right walking shoes. First of all, not all sneakers are created the same. Shoes optimal for walking and shoes optimal for running differ. Think about the workouts themselves. When you run, your feet are taking equal turns leaving the ground. When you walk, one foot is always touching the ground. Therefore, the amount of pounding is not comparable. When you run, up to three or four times your body weight is impacting the ground, whereas walking causes you to strike with the impact of only one and a half times your weight.

This is one reason why runners can develop knee problems more than any other injury. The extra weight jolting the knees from all the strike pressure can cause a lot of wear and tear. Eventually, the knee can break down. I've been blessed to never have knee problems, even while running marathons. But the truth is, I have carried around so much extra weight in my lifetime, and now lost it, that my knees aren't affected by the extra pressure of the pounding. In other words, my frame is already conditioned for added stress. However, the same excess pounds that have helped me avoid knee injuries have caused me to have ankle, Achilles, and feet issues today. Go figure.

Remember in the first chapter, I told you why I walk. I want to help you have the best information possible to avoid unnecessary pain and injury that has the potential to keep you off the highway to healthy living!

Before you go shopping, take a moment at home to grab an old pair of your sneakers. Check out the bottoms. The heel, to be exact. Notice if there is even wear on the rubber, or if the inner or outer edges seem to be more worn. Note: This is the only piece of information you should take with you from home (other than this book, of course). Now, notice I didn't say you should be getting ready to go shopping in front of your computer. Shopping for your first proper walking shoes should be done in person. It's important you figure out which shoes work best for you, and then you can feel free to look for the best deal!

So you've arrived at the store; what do you do next? Well, what you don't do is ask the eighteen-year-old kid working there to help you pick out a pretty pair on sale. Remember, you are the one who will be wearing them and dealing with the repercussions of a haphazard choice. He might be working at Burger King by the time you figure out he had no clue what you needed.

There is a simple test you can give to your potential footwear, but before you conduct it, remember the information from home.

If your shoe was worn evenly, you likely have a neutral foot. This means whenever you strike down, your gait, the way you move through the motion, is basically even as well. The shoes you begin looking at should have the same amount of support on the inside of the heel as they do on the outside. Now, if your shoe was more worn on the outer edges, you are an underpronator. Your heel tends to not make it totally over whenever you strike down. This means look for shoes that have a little bit of a buildup on the inside edge to balance your heel strike. Now, if after taking a peek at the bottom of your shoe, it is more worn on the inner edges, you are officially an overpronator. This means your foot tends to roll all the way over whenever you strike . . . you'll need to look for a shoe with more buildup on the outer edges.

Now that you have narrowed it down to a few pair that fit your gait, it's time for you to do my "Bend, twist, tap, and rock" test:

Bend: A good walking shoe should bend. When you hold up the shoe from behind, you should be able to push up on the toe box. Think about what happens when you are walking. You push down on the ball of your foot, just before you lift it. Therefore, without some give, the front of your foot will be fighting to lift every step, without the flexibility to do it.

Twist: Because your foot will be striking and then bending, it's important your shoe has a bit of flexibility with a twisting motion. Simply grab your potential purchase from the front and back and twist to cause some forced resistance. If there is no give, you don't want this shoe. The shoe needs to be able to "take" a small twist.

Tap: Trust me, you don't want to be fighting with your shoes every step of the way. The best walking shoes will have a low, rounded heel. This way as you strike, with ease, it will lift the front of your foot. To do the tap test, put the potential shoe on the ground and then firmly place a pen or a pencil inside the back of the shoe. If the front lifts off the ground, good! If it doesn't, pass on them.

Rock: Okay. Don't laugh. This is the only part of the test that's really negotiable. Chances are you're not going to wear your walking shoes in a fashion show. I get that! However, I'm a firm believer in the ROCK test. This means, can you "rock" them? In other words, they don't need to be beautiful and match your entire exercise wardrobe, but will you cringe every time you put them on? Or can you feel presentable in them? If you have absolutely no fashion sense, care, or concern, skip this whole thing. But if putting on these puppies you're considering makes you feel like you're sporting the equivalent to Ronald McDonald's red shoes, keep shopping. There are too many shoe choices out there to settle for a pair that will make you feel like a clown!

So now you hopefully have it narrowed down to a few pairs of shoes. It's time to ask for a size. This can vary a lot depending on the manufacturer, and most people find getting a half size bigger than they measure makes the most sense. This accommodates for the potential swelling that takes place during exercise. Here's a tip: once you lace up your walking shoes, you should be able to press your thumb down in the front and barely feel the tip of your toe.

Now I know I haven't discussed the topic of cost and money. I'm a woman, what do you expect? But I'm not naïve when it comes to being on a budget (at least, I'm working on it regularly, for my husband's sake). There are a few things I will say about this subject. Shoes are the only real investment you are making in your road to becoming more fit. This means sacrificing in other areas to have a proper pair is worth it.

Of course, I'm not saying to tell the electric company folks that shoes seemed more important this week than power. However, you can be a savvy shopper. Go out and look, figure out what shoes you need, and then go home and look online for the same shoes at a lower price. Or better yet, see if the store you found them at is willing to price-match. This way, if you find them cheaper on the internet (and you likely will), ask if they will accept a computer printout to verify the cost and then allow you to pay the lower price. This is a great way to avoid having to wait for and pay for shipping. And most stores would rather have your money, even if it means they'll be making a little less profit.

Basically, I really don't care which store you decide to buy from. I just don't want you to fill up your bank of excuses because you wasted money on the wrong shoes and have decided it is too painful to walk. It's a good thing I'm shy about how I feel, huh? Happy shoe shopping! It probably won't be the most beautiful pair you'll ever buy, but trust me, they have the most potential to make you feel like a million bucks!

Part 2

The How

7

Walk with a Sweet Swagger

*M*oving from God's acceptance to desiring to be more acceptable is meant to be a lifelong journey of walking with Him spiritually, emotionally, and physically. Once you have recognized the desire, faith will help you stay the course. Towards the end of the book I'll address this in greater detail.

There is no way to get anywhere spectacular without believing it's worth the trip. Therefore, having confidence while you're walking is important. I like to call it possessing a sweet swagger! We are not rigged to be "perfect walkers" on our own. Yet we have just established God wants us to work on achieving perfection all the time, regardless.

Most people don't believe any measurement of perfection is possible. They waste a lot of time naming and claiming their struggles instead of naming and claiming the power of God to help them have victory. The resurrection of Christ guarantees all of His children the power to pursue higher levels of perfection every day. However, successes are guaranteed only if we are willing to seek perfection that is according to His standards, not anyone else's. A prayer to have increased faith in His perfect timing is also critical.

One of the reasons we have trouble with this kind of faith is due to a lack of patience and willingness to let Him lead. God won't force His ability to help us get there. I can remember trying to have a special afternoon with my son Jake. He was around three years old. The plan was to stop off at Wal-Mart for a few things I needed, for him. Next, we were going to get some ice cream. After, we had a play date at the park with his friends. When we got to the store, I decided to let him walk beside me instead of putting him in the stroller. Not only was he getting too big for it, he was also pretty sure he was too cool to be seen in it. The issue we had began about two minutes after we set off down the aisles. His three-year-old patience bank ran out. In fact, I think it was overdrawn. He began knocking stuff off all the shelves. No matter what I said to threaten him and let him know he was in imminent jeopardy of forgoing the rest of our big afternoon plans, it didn't matter. Both the ice cream and play date must have seemed like distant dreams, because he continued to behave like a little brat.

I became so aggravated. Here I wanted to buy some things for him (you know, the usual: pull-ups, Teddy-grahams, and some bubbles) and then take him to have some ice cream. And after that, I was also going to let him run around with his buddies. And he blew it! After a few warnings, I gently grabbed his hand and walked him out to our car, where I strapped him in his booster seat and drove him back to our house. We entered our home with nothing to show for our afternoon but tears from us both. Being a good parent meant I had to show him that, by leaving, I refused to reward him for not listening! Being a great parent meant giving him the space to make the choice, while I maintained the willingness to let him try again tomorrow.

Do you think we are ever guilty of acting like a three-year-old when it comes to our sin and struggles? We have God offering to lead us and give us so much, and instead we regularly stop and throw temper tantrums. *But God, I'm tired. But God, this isn't fun. But God, I'm bored. But God,* (and this one is the best) *are we there yet?* He listens. He leads. He even lets us complain. Yet in His mercy, He eventually takes us exactly back to where we started. And it's not because He wants us to be angry at Him or sad about our circumstances. It's that He wants us to trust the system of sacrificial living. All rewards are subject to sacrifice. If not, why did God need to send His only Son to suffer on a cross? Have you ever thrown a fit because you didn't like the timing or direction God was taking you in? Or maybe you've lacked belief in His competence to get you where you need to be.

I was about to teach a spin class when my cell phone rang. On the line was my husband, Keith. "Babe," he said. "I'm on the golf course and I'm having some serious pain. It's in my stomach. I've never felt anything like this; what should I do?" Well, I was clueless as to what was going on. So I told him to head to the hospital and I'd meet him there. After a battery of tests, the emergency room doctor said Keith's gall bladder needed to come out. This was the first time he was going to have anesthesia or surgery. He was a wreck. Well, we signed the okay for him to be put under and have the infected part of his body removed.

Imagine if next, a man had walked in wearing a white doctor coat completely unbuttoned so we could read his "I Love New York" T-shirt, carrying a large butcher knife, sporting a Yankees baseball cap—and then he said "Hi, y'all, are we ready to remove that kidney or what?"

Can you say, bye-bye hospital, hello pain?

The only way to walk with God is to trust Him entirely. You must know that even if your faith is similar to a three-year-old's, He still has big plans for you. Even if you're in tremendous pain emotionally, He is the only doctor fully capable of doing the surgery to fix you, your body, and your life. Faith is the only special equipment you need to begin walking with a sweet swagger. Faith that God's taking you somewhere special, and faith He can fix any part of you that breaks along the way.

Every day when you wake up and surrender your body to Him, the road to wellness begins. Notice I said every day. Not just the day you walk down the aisle and say a prayer of repentance, or the day you step on a scale and decide enough is enough. This is the most freeing way you could possibly look at long-term fitness and weight maintenance. Here's the best part: your ultimate journey to wellness will be completed when you get a heavenly body. This marks the end of the road to becoming acceptable, and commences the path to your perfection. Freedom from the struggle will cease. When you think about it, taking "before and after" photos seems pretty silly.

Now it's time to talk about how to begin walking with Him. First of all, before your feet even hit the floor in the morning, pray and ask Him to help you schedule your day with enough time to go for a physical walk. And then request His guidance to help you choose healthy meals. Why not ask

Him for the strength to say no to temptation (i.e., cheesecake for dessert on a Monday) and ask Him for the peace to say yes to an occasional pleasure (i.e., chocolate—anytime!) I imagine the diet industry would begin to suffer and sneaker manufacturers would begin to run out of rubber if you'd take this approach to health and fitness.

Now when I say go out for a physical walk, I do mean in the traditional sense. You know, the act of creating movement with your arms and legs. In case you're wondering, I agree: it shouldn't take an entire book to explain "how to walk," either. (And if I can do it, look for my next book to be on "breathing.") However, I am going to help you learn to maximize the most natural form of exercise on the planet.

This book will be your guide to utilizing walking as a super-highway to heaven, while becoming super-fit! I will tell you this: I have never found another workout to be comparable. Walking not only trains your body, but it also renews your mind, and has the power to reignite your relationship with God, each and every time.

But before you hit the road, you'll need to take a risk. I remember back to just after I finished writing my first book, *Never Say Diet*. For a few days prior to the deadline, I dreaded clicking "send" on the file. It seriously gave me heart palpitations. It felt like I was handing over my soul in a Word document. After I finally "sent" it, eventually it came back a few weeks later. But this time the file had a new name, "revised." Honestly, when I opened it up for the first time, I was pretty convinced a two-year-old would try harder to repaint a Picasso than my editor would try to protect "my words." Wow, was I wrong!

You see friends, here's the shocking truth: you can't get better at anything without risking revision. Yes, the act of walking can deepen your relationship with God and do many more things for your life; however, you'll need to risk revising your old perceptions when it comes to how to walk in the three areas of faith, food, and fitness. How do you see yourself? Are some foods from the enemy? And what is the real reason to exercise? Don't worry; I'm going to help you discover the answers to them all.

With all this hype, you may be thinking, *Seriously, Chantel? What kind of walking are we talking about?* I know. This sounds like some serious new benefits from something many of us have been doing since before we could form a sentence. For the record: walking is the simplest, cheapest, and most basic form of exercise. Its power is often downplayed or chalked off. Do you realize every time you go out for a walk, no matter where you are, you have the creator of the concept, the equipment, and the fuel desiring to hang out with you the whole time? And for no charge. Imagine if Thomas Edison came over every time a lightbulb went out in your home. And each time he showed up, he coached you on how to install a new one while he retold the "how I dreamed up the electric light" story with real tears in his eyes. Trust me, you would never get bored by it. Next, magnify this scenario about a million times. This is what I have found walking with God feels like. And so will you.

It's incredible to think about Him engineering our limbs to move back and forth and create energy. Plus, it can be done today, without having to wait for rush shipping and handling. Not only will walking take you places, literally, it also has the power to burn off a bagel. I imagine you're ready to throw on your sneakers. But after the chapter on shoes, you're not even sure you have the right ones. Relax! I'm here to hang out with you along the way and to answer many of your concerns, such as proper nutrition for losing weight, as well as what amount of intensity works best, and when. But for now, all you really need to decide is that you are willing to let me show you how to begin walking stronger than ever before, and that you're going to have fun doing it.

If you are, get ready. But first, this kind of walking will begin with one small detour. Yes, I know, you haven't even hit the road yet. But what I'm talking about here is where you're trying to get to. Initially, you'll need to put away any form of measuring. This means a watch, a scale, a GPS—you get the idea. Time, weight loss, and distance are not your primary goals. Yet. And don't even think about trying to multitask, either. In other words, your walking workouts won't be the perfect opportunity to learn French on your iPod with Rosetta Stone. However, I did say, "this kind of walking begins with . . ." I didn't say you won't walk strong for long periods of time, experience major weight loss, train for a 5K sometime soon, or perhaps even learn a new language if you really want to. But truly learning to walk strong and effectively happens only when you begin by ditching desires that are based on an external reward. In other words, let longer workouts, better-fitting pants, and greater distances traveled be awesome by-products, not driving motives.

The word *swagger* is indicative of walking with confidence or pride. However, when you have a sweet swagger, you are doing it with humility, and your pride is coming from the confidence you have in your leader. Trust me, no team would ever win a championship if they didn't trust their coach to take them there. But because they do, they can run onto the field with their hands up in the air.

Begin each and every workout and walk knowing God is in front of you, beside you, and behind you at all times. This means no fear you won't finish. No worry you won't be able to keep up. And no sadness if you can't go as long as you were hoping to go, due to other obligations.

It's time to get walking with a sweet swagger.

To kick off your Walk with Him program, go out for one 30-minute walk. That's it! A simple, straightforward walk. Don't worry about fancy equipment, or even matching clothes for that matter. Just go out the door, head in one direction for 15 minutes, and turn around. Don't wait for a cloudless sky or a gentle breeze—just get up and go! Also, it's important not to worry about your level of intensity, either. You can't be competitive until you're consistent.

During this first walk, go out and spend the first 15 minutes saying aloud what you're most thankful for. You know, count your blessings!

For the second half of your walk, pray using these areas, the five Fs, as your guideline. You'll want to personalize your prayers to match your life, needs, and concerns.

Forgiveness	Thank God for forgiving your sin
Family	Bring Him your family concerns
Friends	Give Him your friendships and ask for His blessing
Finances	Seek wisdom and guidance
Faithfulness	Ask Him to help you "walk the walk"

You will find me referring to each of these areas many times in this book. They represent the full gamut of our lives.

Where I went for my first walk with God:

_____

_____

I thanked Him for:

_____

_____

_____

I prayed for:

_____

_____

_____

I feel:

_____

_____

_____

8

We Need a Month

*N*ow that your first walk is behind you, it's time to get to work. We need a month. Before you agree (and it is up to you), you need to know a few things. First of all, "we" is "God and I." God and myself. In this book, we are a tag team, introducing you to the power of walking. But here's why we need a month.

I've said it many times already: walking with Him is the journey of a lifetime. I'm talking in terms of learning the unforced rhythms of grace and continuing to do so for as long as you are alive. However, there is a systematic way you can approach walking with Him each time that will revive and renew you regularly. And you can learn it in a month! This essentially means that, going forward, you'll have a tried-and-true plan for maintaining the balance of healthy living—physically, mentally, and spiritually.

Let's talk about the span of a month. I could have certainly said "Give me a year." But the truth is, while you'll want God walking with you year-round, you'd get tired of me! Then I thought about ninety days. This seems to be a pretty common timetable for many programs. But as I really looked at what you need to know and how long it would take me to tell it to you, a month was perfect.

A month is a special measurement of time. I'm sure you realize a calendar is broken down into months. But do you know why? It's because a month is approximately the number of days it takes the moon to circle the earth. Not only does the moon's location in this process affect the tides and fishing, it also affects our minds and bodies. It's no secret people can tend to be a little crazy when there's a full moon!

God created a woman's body to have a monthlong cycle of menstruation. You have probably noticed (and if you haven't, trust me, someone in your life has) there is a wide range of things happening and changing from week to week for us, ladies. This process gives our bodies the opportunity to prepare for conception, or new life, regularly.

I want you to be able to use this Walk with Him program for the rest of your life. However, realistically I know life is a series of high tides and low tides. Once you learn this system of how to walk strong physically, emotionally, and spiritually, no matter where you find yourself in the sea of life, you'll be able to dive back in!

Here is a brief description of the four weeks:

Week One   Just for Fun
Week Two   Find Your Groove
Week Three Get More Peace
Week Four   It's Time for More

Week One: Just for Fun

The first week of your Walk with Him journey is going to be, plainly and simply, fun! Do you know most people don't smile enough? There are forty-four muscles in your face. Our God has designed our faces to show expressions. It actually takes far less energy and fewer muscles to smile than it does to create an angry face. God is into energy conservation, folks. Which expression do you think we should be doing more of?

Here are some reasons for you to learn how to smile more while you walk with Him:

A smile draws people in.
When we see someone smiling, we all want to know: what's so funny?
A smile can change a mood.
Try screaming at someone with a grin on your face. It's not easy, is it?
A smile is contagious.
Smile and others smile back. But would you frown back at someone?
A smile makes you look younger.
Raise the corners of your mouth and see an instant face-lift!
A smile is relaxing.
A smile lowers blood pressure and forces tension to leave your face.
A smile is energizing.
A smile is the international symbol for joy and happiness.

While there are some technical things about walking I will talk about shortly, you must first enjoy it. No matter how good you are at something, or how many benefits it has, if you don't find pleasure from it you'll become aggravated, resentful, and quit! Week one you will fall in love with walking.

Week Two: Find Your Groove

"Groove." I think this word from the 1970s is cool.

Finding your groove sounds personal yet productive, right? Moving into week two, we'll be walking with Him but focusing a lot on what makes you unique. This means you'll be discovering some of your glitches when it comes to why you are who you are, and why you have struggled in some areas while soaring in others.

Finding your groove is going to help you get over those humps when they come up. You see, getting some enthusiasm to start something new isn't all that hard, especially if depression and misery are present from the get-go. But maintaining a long-term fitness plan is another story. The only way to make this happen is to have a personal program. Recall the story of Cheryl and how she accomplished walking a half marathon? If she had tried to make her groove match anyone else's on the team, she would have quit long before race day.

In week two, you'll learn more about your fitness level and what it means to push its boundaries. We'll take a test to figure out where you're the strongest and where there is room for improvement. The greatest benefit from week two is personal empowerment. When someone walks into a gym after a hiatus, there is a natural tendency to try to keep up with other "gym rats." Often feelings of failure can swallow up good intentions and sabotage righteous efforts. The option of giving up will be out the door after this week.

Week Three: Get More Peace

Got peace? Before you answer, I'm sure we all remember the famous "Got Milk?" advertising campaign from back in the mid-90s. It was one of the corporate masterminds at Goodby, Silverstein & Partners advertising agency who came up with it. He had the idea that if he utilized a deprivation strategy, more milk would sell. The first ads featured a chocolate chip cookie, a brownie, or a cupcake with a few bites missing, and the words "Got Milk?" The agency decided by implying the need for milk as a perfect complement to a sweet treat, people would begin to buy more and drink more.

It not only worked, it became one of the most notable advertising campaigns of all time. And it also made milk a "cool drink." A who's who from rock stars to presidents to Olympians has since been photographed sporting the infamous milk mustache.

I'm hoping the third week of your monthlong journey, "Get More Peace," will be a much more effective campaign for you. This week is designed to stir up some deprivation matters of the heart. I think we know having peace is a good thing, yet the realization of how to have it despite our circumstances is what most people miss. This week we'll use walking to get more peace!

Week Four: It's Time for More

So now you believe walking is fun, effective, and satisfying, but it must also become challenging to get maximum results!

Week four is all about MORE! Every walk this week will be a lesson in going farther, pushing harder, and becoming better. You wouldn't need my help—or more importantly God's—if you knew how to get better all by yourself. Getting better at anything requires pushing boundaries. Yes, we're focused on the physical benefits of walking; this means there will be some tough challenges the fourth week. But I know your walk with Him also needs depth.

I was at the beach with my kids recently and I had a flashback to my own childhood. I watched a group of children digging in the sand, and one of them said that if they kept on going, they'd eventually get to see China! I remembered hearing and saying the same thing back when I played with my friends in the dirt. Sadly, not once did we get there! But we sure kept on digging for many days, hoping we eventually would.

The only way to get anywhere good is to keep on believing you're almost there, and when you do this, you may find the process of getting there can be better than your arrival. On earth, none of us will truly ever walk with God all the time. It's impossible for many reasons. But approaching each area of our fitness with the hope we're almost there is critical. The truth is, every day we walk with the Lord, we are a little bit closer to eternity!

I've already told you the importance of having proper footwear. Now I want to encourage you to have a stopwatch, or at least a watch that is sweat-proof, to wear. You will start by measuring your walks in terms of time. Here's why: distance is not a level playing field. What if you live in a mountainous region and someone else lives at sea level? Sure, eventually, knowing exactly how far you're going can be good information. But it doesn't make sense to use distance as a starting point. How far you can go will fluctuate on a given day, and it also limits you to the same route. However, the number of minutes you go out and walk is entirely straightforward. Therefore, all your walking workouts for the first four weeks have time guidelines.

As far as weather challenges and treadmills go, here's what I'll say: I personally enjoy using a treadmill sometimes. But it can be much more difficult to tune out noise and truly walk with Him this way. However, it can be done; I've done it. Due to rain or travel, and many other factors, I've used a gym for my walking workouts many times. To sum it up: there is serious beauty in nature, while always walking on a conveyer belt can be seriously distracting.

We will not focus much on intensity or speed the first week. However, along the way, I will be talking more about both. You will also find, for each of the four weeks, there is a prescription for the number of days for you to walk as well as a planned amount of time for you to spend doing it. It's important that you choose the time of day and days that work best for you. However, if by the middle of week two you have already missed a day, do yourself a favor and begin again at week one. You need to know that consistency is key at this point. If you don't invest the full amount of time into this month, you may compromise your long-term success. While a little extra won't hurt, missing days along the way will.

Before we get into the Walk with Him program, I want to share three stretches with you. You should plan to use all of them regularly to stay injury-free. In addition, they will make your recovery time between walks shorter. Try them now, if you'd like; however, also plan to use them before and after your regular walks.

Later in the book, we'll get more in-depth when it comes to stretching. For an instructional video for each of these stretches, visit my website, www.faithfoodfitness.com.

Chin Up

Standing straight, with your feet shoulder-width apart, interlace your fingers in front of you. Next, press your arms and hands away from your body, palms out, and reach them up as far as you can. When your hands are directly overhead, slowly drop your head all the way back, relaxing your neck and bringing your chin up toward the ceiling as far as it will go. Hold for 20 seconds.

Next, keeping your chin up, rotate your upper body toward your right side, still reaching up. Hold for 20 seconds. Switch to the left side, and hold for another 20 seconds.

Bow Down

Standing straight, with your feet slightly wider than shoulder-width apart, lift your arms in front of you until they are parallel with your shoulders. Next, lower your chin to your chest. Now, begin to bend at your waist, keeping your back rounded and your pelvis tucked. Do this until you feel a pulling stretch in the back of your legs (hamstrings) and your lower back as well (lumbar spine). Do not lock your knees. You may lower your arms if needed. Hold for 15 seconds. Break. Hold for 20 seconds. Break. Hold for 30 seconds.

Chair Squat

Now, standing straight with your feet slightly wider than shoulder-width apart, reach your arms straight up, with palms facing in, and lower your body as if you were going to sit in a chair. Hold. Your weight should be in your heels. Try wiggling your toes to make sure. The key to this exercise is enduring the burning in the thighs (quadriceps).

Work your way up to holding this position for 30 seconds. Initially, start with just 15 seconds.

Walk with Him, Week One

Just for Fun

Here we go!

Now, I'm not one of those women who thinks of being pregnant as fun. Not even a little bit. Number one, it's basically a science experiment going on inside my body. Number two, I don't find it fun to try to control my bladder and my emotions at the same time. And it's really not fun to be asked if you're having twins when you're only four months along with one baby!

However, I do think having a baby is a total blast! Have I confused you? Let me clarify. It's not the actual process I like, but it's every moment thereafter. I seriously love all parts of those first few weeks, getting to know the little person who has just entered our lives. From the first feeding to the first bath, to the first time she slept for three hours during the night, it's all fun . . . at least to me.

But don't worry. I'm not naïve. I've put in my time at the park, on the playground, hanging out with some of you who couldn't agree less! You think pregnancy is awesome, but that first couple of weeks is the worst. Whether it's trying to recognize "which cry" it is or wondering if she is getting enough to eat, it's all a frustrating guessing game to you. Of course you love your baby; you just don't like some parts of the initial process. It's not fun, to you.

What You Need to Know: Week One

Whether or not we are on the same page when it comes to how we define fun isn't important. What is important is knowing how and why to have fun while walking this week. You see, if you find a way to have fun doing something, you'll find a way to do it more often. Maybe that's why I have four kids . . . my husband and I have both found out how to have fun in the process!

For me, the beginning of becoming a walker required familiar music with a major beat to it. I happen to love all gospel music and lots of drums, like you'll find in African music. For you, however, it may be more fun for you not to have any music on at all. I even know a woman who planned her walks as time to catch up with her oldest and dearest friend, who lived in another state. She just wore an earpiece connected to her cell phone. I imagine they both had a blast as long as her friend knew it was her calling, and not some heavy-breathing prankster.

I'm sure you get the basic idea. Fun is relative but critical!

What are some ways you could make walking fun?

_____

_____

Walk with Him: Week One Plan

Three walks, 30 minutes each

You will be walking three days this first week and for a total of 30 minutes each day. Plan to wear something comfortable, along with your well-fitted shoes. Also, be sure to have lots of water to drink before you go out. Decide ahead of time which direction you'll head. All three walks this week will have a different theme designed to help you focus on having fun. They are laughter, joy, and reward.

Week One—Walk One—Day/Date: _____

30 minutes

Pre-Walk Challenge: Learn the Joy of Laughter

I laugh at silly stuff. In fact, some of my favorite things to laugh about are things my kids have said, or stuff I've seen people do that makes no sense to me. Like the time I watched two people get in a heated argument over a front row parking space at the gym. Plus, there was another space open just a few feet away. Think about it: both people are going inside the place to exercise. Would a few extra steps really matter?

Use this 30 minutes to recall at least five moments of laughter in your life. Be ready to list a few of them when you return. It can be a movie, a food incident, or the time you left church and forgot to pick up your child from the nursery (or am I the only one who's done this?).

Notice exactly what time it is as you set out for this walk. And calculate what the time will be in 15 minutes. This will be your turnaround point. Now get going! Also pay attention to your facial expressions as you begin to move. Whenever someone catches your eye along the way, flash them a friendly smile. (Friendly, ladies, not flirty. There is a major difference.) Usually including a little nod helps. And one more thing: when it comes to how fast you're walking, don't focus too much on your speed this week. Be sure to keep a steady and challenging pace and try to keep it consistent for now.

Go have fun!

Post-Walk Chat

So you're back—and you've walked for 30 minutes, and hopefully had a few laughs.

What was so funny, anyway?

_____

_____

_____

Week One—Walk Two—Day/Date: _____

30 minutes

Pre-Walk Challenge: Joy to the World

You're probably not reading this anywhere near Christmas. But just for this one walk, we're going to pretend it's the holiday season. One of the most familiar carols of all time is "Joy to the World."

You know the words:

> Joy to the world, the Lord is come!
> Let earth receive her King;

Let every heart prepare Him room,
And heaven and nature sing,
And heaven and nature sing,
And heaven, and heaven, and nature sing.

This walk will also be 30 minutes, and once again you should set a turnaround time before you head out. But this time, I want you to plan on saying or singing these lyrics at least five times during your walk. I know it may sound a little corny, but I'll take the risk of you thinking I'm cheesy. Because I know when we sing these words there is no way we can feel down. Plus, there's a nice rhythm to the song that makes you want to move your arms and march.

Also, you should use this walk to define things in your life that have brought you joy, lately. Joy can be defined as "extreme happiness." Note the key word: lately. The joy you once got from your child's straight-A report card may have been swallowed up by a recent string of Cs. So don't focus so much on fleeting joys. For example, I have found regular joy in cooking with my children—from their silly antics, to creating a menu, to the way my sons Jake and Luke compete in creating the fanciest plate with their green beans sticking in hills of mashed potatoes. Take time today to recall joy you've found in recent memories. Also consider the eternal joy heaven has offered us all, the real joy to the world.

Post-Walk Chat

What were your joyful thoughts about today?

_____

_____

_____

Do you think having joy is a choice?

_____

_____

_____

What are some things you could plan to do in the next three days to bring someone else joy?

_____

_____

_____

Week One—Walk Three—Day/Date: _____

30 minutes

Pre-Walk Challenge: Reaping Rewards

The fun of sacrifice comes in the form of rewards. It's more fun to do anything when you know there is a potential celebration waiting for you. My daughter wouldn't have taken her driving test three times unless she believed it would be awesome to have some freedom. In fact, each time she was told she didn't pass, it got funnier to both of us. For her, the excitement took over her aggravation. For me, the excitement she was still a passenger made me happy. Use your 30-minute walk today to think about the rewards waiting for you in a month. You are going to have a great time today. Use today's walk to come up with one specific way you will celebrate at the end of this four-week period. Even if you are using the program for the third or fourth time, don't skip this. A reward system will help you stay focused.

Post-Walk Chat

What rewards are you looking for over the next four weeks?

_____

_____

_____

How will you celebrate?

_____

_____

_____

Looking beyond the next four weeks, where do you see yourself in a year in terms of wellness?

_____

_____

_____

10

Walk with Him, Week Two

Find Your Groove

There is no way you will excel at anything without putting your ego on the line. One of the most perfect examples I've seen of this happens regularly on a television show called *Top Chef: Masters*. This program is a spin-off of the Emmy Award–winning show *Top Chef*. But on this one, well-known seasoned chefs from around the world arrive to compete with one another. There is no question about whether they are entirely capable; after all, they have been chosen based upon their proven success. Instead, it's a matter of a panel of judges interpreting whose food tastes the best on a specific day. After watching it many times, I know the secret. It all comes down to *groove*. When one of these chefs is in their groove—for example, they own a seafood restaurant and the challenge is to make a creative shrimp dish—they end up doing quite well. However, when the chef isn't in their groove—such as they've been asked to make a pie, but they know how to make only apple pie without a recipe and apples aren't available—watch out. Butter and pans will be flying.

The importance of finding your groove while walking with God comes down to creating a comfort level and defining areas for future improvement. You obviously know how to walk. And you also have already put in some time walking. Now, you're going to discover where you are strongest and where you feel weak.

This week you'll be going out three times for three walks, again. However, the first will be 30 minutes. The second will be 45 minutes, and the third one will be for an hour. Don't be intimidated by the longer walking times. Your walking program needs to help you move past your fears that you're not able, and help you trust your Creator to give you supernatural strength and endurance. From now on, each of the week's walking workouts will contain a Walk with Him challenge. Be sure to read these first, so you know what to do during your walk. Also, take a few moments to read the Bible passage that follows. As you head out for your walk, before you power up an iPod or some other noise, spend a few moments thinking about the deeper meaning of the Scripture. When you return, reread the Scripture passage and answer the spiritual and physical fitness focus questions.

Also: don't forget to do the three stretches you have already learned before each workout.

Walk with Him: Week Two Plan

Three walks: 30 minutes, 45 minutes, and 60 minutes

Week Two—Walk One—Day/Date: _____

30 minutes

Pre-Walk Challenge

As you head out for this walk, take an altogether new route than you have in the past. If you are going to the gym, get on a treadmill you've never stepped on. Now, take a look at your watch. For every 4 minutes you are walking at a steady pace, pick up your pace for 1 minute straight. This minute should cause you to get a little out of breath. Also, it will be important to turn around at minute 15 and head back home.

Read Mark 2:1–12:

> When Jesus returned to Capernaum several days later, the news spread quickly that he was back home. Soon the house where he was staying was so packed with visitors that there was no more room, even outside the door. While he was preaching God's word to them, four men arrived carrying a paralyzed man on a mat. They couldn't bring him to Jesus because of the crowd, so they dug a hole through the roof above his head. Then they lowered the man on his mat, right down in front of Jesus. Seeing their faith, Jesus said to the paralyzed man, "My child, your sins are forgiven."
>
> But some of the teachers of religious law who were sitting there thought to themselves, "What is he saying? This is blasphemy! Only God can forgive sins!"
>
> Jesus knew immediately what they were thinking, so he asked them, "Why do you question this in your hearts? Is it easier to say to the paralyzed man 'Your sins are forgiven,' or 'Stand up, pick up your mat, and walk'? So I will prove to you that the Son of Man has the authority on earth to forgive sins." Then Jesus turned to the paralyzed man and said, "Stand up, pick up your mat, and go home!"
>
> And the man jumped up, grabbed his mat, and walked out through the stunned onlookers. They were all amazed and

praised God, exclaiming, "We've never seen anything like this before!" (NLT)

Think about this verse as you head out, and have a beautiful walk!

Post-Walk Chat

Be honest. Were you a little annoyed when I told you to go a new route, or get on a new treadmill, for this workout?

_____

_____

Did you find it difficult to push yourself for 1 minute out of every 5?

_____

Were you able to go immediately back to your steady pace after each fast minute was over, or did you need to slow down considerably?

_____

At the end of your workout, did you feel more "spent" than you had after past workouts?

_____

The purpose of today's physical challenge was to test your "groove" when it comes to being uncomfortable. If you welcomed the switch-up, and had your best walking workout yet, your "groove" is likely to be in full force when you are able to be competitive, even if it's just with yourself. Be willing to use this to go farther and challenge others to follow. Now, if you found yourself missing your old route, and were not really any more motivated, although you did well and completed the challenge you probably get into your "groove" best when you feel safe and comfortable. This is not a bad thing. Just be sure that you don't choose comfort over personal growth.

The passage in Mark 2 was about the power of Jesus not only to forgive sin, but to heal.

Besides the paralyzed man, whose faith was on the line?

_____

_____

_____

_____

Why do you think Jesus made the statement, "Your sins are forgiven," to the sick man, instead of simply healing him?

_____

_____

_____

_____

Do you think we often underestimate God's power to heal our minor stuff because we think He's too busy with big stuff, or because we just don't believe He can?

_____

_____

_____

What are you asking Him to heal at this time?

_____

_____

_____

Week Two—Walk Two—Day/Date: _____

45 minutes

Pre-Walk Challenge

As you head out for your first longer walk today, plan on using this time to go shopping—but only in your mind! For the first 5 minutes, begin to think of something you would buy if you had $500 dollars earmarked just for you. This means no other bills, other obligations, or new shoes for the kids can come out of it. Keep at a steady pace for the following 30 minutes. Be sure to turn around at about 20–25 minutes into the walk. As you come up to the last 10 minutes, try to increase your speed enough to raise your heart rate, but not so much as to become entirely out of breath.

Read Ephesians 2:4–10:

> It wasn't so long ago that you were mired in that old stagnant life of sin. You let the world, which doesn't know the first thing about living, tell you how to live. You filled your lungs with polluted unbelief, and then exhaled disobedience. We all did it, all of us doing what we felt like doing, when we felt like doing it, all of us in the same boat. It's a wonder God didn't lose his temper and do away with the whole lot of us. Instead, immense in mercy and with an incredible love, he embraced us. He took our sin-dead lives and made us alive in Christ. He did all this on his own, with no help from us! Then he picked us up and set us down in highest heaven in company with Jesus, our Messiah.

Now God has us where he wants us, with all the time in this world and the next to shower grace and kindness upon us in Christ Jesus. Saving is all his idea, and all his work. All we do is trust him enough to let him do it. It's God's gift from start to finish! We don't play the major role. If we did, we'd probably go around bragging that we'd done the whole thing! No, we neither make nor save ourselves. God does both the making and saving. He creates each of us by Christ Jesus to join him in the work he does, the good work he has gotten ready for us to do, work we had better be doing. (Message)

Time to hit the road.

Post-Walk Chat

Did you get excited when I said the word *shopping*?

_____

Did you have trouble thinking of something for only yourself?

_____

Was what you chose practical or frivolous?

_____

What was your favorite part of the walk—the first 35 minutes, or the last 10?

_____

The purpose of today's Walk with Him challenge was to see if you could get into the "groove" of taking care of yourself first. You see, many people are so wired to think of everyone else, they forget that having energy for others happens only if you make regular deposits into your own bank of wellness. If you had a lot of trouble coming up with something you'd buy for only you, don't worry. You "groove" best when doing for others. While this is an awesome way to live, you won't have as much to give if you don't take time for yourself. On the other hand, if you had no trouble whatsoever coming up with a long list, your "groove" is entirely different. You need to focus on priorities. This means take good care of you—and then move on to others.

The passage in Ephesians was a reminder of God's mercy to us.

What is your definition of mercy?

_____

_____

Why do you think we try to take so much credit when we are good?

_____

_____

_____

If God does the creating and the saving, do you think we should relax a little more and let Him be in charge?

_____

_____

_____

In what areas do you need to relax more?

_____

_____

Week Two—Walk Three—Day/Date: _____

60 minutes

Pre-Walk Challenge

You and I both have 24 hours in a day. This doesn't fluctuate for either of us. Today's walk is going to account for 1/24th of your day. NO BIG DEAL! Your walk today is going to be broken down into four quarters, or four 15-minute segments. For the first quarter, just go out and have fun, sing, listen to music, get warmed up. The second quarter is time to get more serious. Think of two people in your life who are hurting and some ways you could cheer them up. Now you're halfway through, so you'll want to turn back around. For the third quarter, it's family time. Spend these minutes praying for your family and thanking God for each member. And for the final quarter, turn the noise back up, sing, or whatever, and give everything you've got for a high-energy finish.

Read 2 Corinthians 5:6–10:

> Therefore we are always confident and know that as long as we are at home in the body we are away from the Lord. For we live by faith, not by sight. We are confident, I say, and would prefer to be away from the body and at home with the Lord. So we make it our goal to please him, whether we are at home in the body or away from it. For we must all appear before the judgment seat of Christ, so that each of us may receive what is due us for the things done while in the body, whether good or bad.

Go out and enjoy your hour-long walk with Him.

Post-Walk Chat

Of all four quarters, which one was your favorite?

_____

What two people are you now planning to bless?

_____

_____

How?

_____

_____

_____

Which family members did you thank God for?

_____

_____

Today's walk was designed to be challenging. If you enjoyed the first or last quarters the most, you most likely get your "groove" on best when you aren't caught up in emotion. You'd rather just "do" than think about it. This means you accomplish a lot but you may tend to hurt other people in the process. Be careful this week to be sensitive to others. Now, if you found the second or third quarters to be your favorite, your "groove" tends to get going when it's focused on helping someone out. The great benefit to your "groove" comfort zone is that you'll not give up quickly if results don't happen fast enough. However, you can also tend to be too relaxed when it comes to making things happen. Seek to find the balance.

Since today's verse talks about our body as not being a permanent home, does this passage mean we shouldn't take care of it?

_____

_____

_____

What does it mean to you to walk by faith, not by sight?

_____

_____

_____

Since the last verse talks about our accountability for actions in the body, do you think this applies to deliberately choosing to do harmful things to our bodies on a regular basis?

_____

_____

_____

Would a diet of pizza, cheeseburgers, fries, and milk shakes seem to apply?

_____

_____

_____

What's the first food you want to thank God for in person?

_____

_____

_____

11

Walk with Him, Week Three

Get More Peace

*T*he theme for week three of the Walk with Him program is peace. Here's the funny part: while attempting to write this chapter, it's been a tremendous challenge for me to try and have any semblance of peace in my life. You name it, it's happened. Keith and I just returned home from an event-filled trip to the mountains. The goal of our vacation was to have some quiet time together while I also got some writing done. While we were away, a tropical storm threatened our house in South Florida (with our children in it!). Then a rattlesnake wandered into the cabin's bathroom. Our last night was also exciting. A black bear decided to wake us up at three in the morning by tossing around trash cans on the porch, perhaps looking for a pre-hibernation snack.

Today, as I try to unpack, I'm sick and am taking a heavy-duty antibiotic. Our family car is broken down, and I just found out it needs a costly repair. On top of everything else, my mother-in-law is recovering from major surgery. Truthfully, if I try to measure how peace-filled I am, at this moment, based on all my life's circumstances, I'd say . . . not so much.

But here's the deal: whether or not you or I have personal peace doesn't need to depend on what's going on in our lives. Our faith is a different story. Remember, faith is something we choose to have based on things we can't see (see Heb. 11). This is why when our lives get crazy our faith can suffer. However, don't let personal peace get mixed up with personal faith. Peace isn't contingent upon our circumstances or us. Even when our faith feels small, peace is readily available to pick up the slack and remind us we can survive. Peace can also protect our faith. The key is to have peace that's not based on our emotional state. When we can begin to live this out, our faith not only deepens, it shows serious authenticity to the rest of the world.

I believe we are all guilty of allowing our emotions and frustrations to rob us of "keeping the faith" or having God's perfect peace. Sometimes life can feel like a game of Monopoly. Our circumstances may make us feel like we're landing in jail regularly. The great news is we all have access to a "get out of jail free" card immediately! You see, the peace God gives us through His Son possesses the power to release us from prison—every time.

Perhaps the most aggravating part of playing Monopoly and landing in jail is the waiting. It's kind of like how life feels when many things are going wrong at once and we still try to manage everything ourselves. Do you understand that we don't need to feel this way, ever? Jesus is an automatic "get out of jail free" card. If you are experiencing a lack of peace, and feel trapped in a prison of pain, there is some good news. Even if your faith feels threatened, peace is always available, and jail can be a place of the past. The cross represents Jesus monopolizing our sin, and handing us a piece of prime real estate—heaven!

In Luke 4:18, Jesus is speaking at the synagogue in Nazareth:

> The Spirit of the Lord is on me,
> because he has anointed me
> to proclaim good news to the poor.
> He has sent me to proclaim freedom for the prisoners
> and recovery of sight for the blind,
> to set the oppressed free.

Notice, He speaks of four groups of people here: the poor, the prisoner, the blind, and the oppressed. There is no one He's left out. Peace and freedom are available for us all. And this past year has taught me this in tremendous ways. My sweet grandfather passed away. My mother became sick and was re-diagnosed with leukemia. Keith and I had some long-time marital issues we tackled. And our fifteen-year-old, Ashley, went on a mission trip to Uganda. All of these trials felt more like a game of trying to balance my emotions and stay out of jail than an opportunity to win a "peace prize." But friends, I can say today that I am able to sincerely thank Him for each one of these things. Looking back on each, I realize I'm really growing up! As I learn to trust God and walk closer with Him, I've become totally dependent on Him. I'm convinced peace has taken on a deeper meaning in my life because these things have happened, not despite them!

Dependence on God our Father is nothing like real-life parenting. As moms and dads, we aim to raise children who are independent of us. It's because we know we won't be around forever to care for them. But do you realize that utter peace comes from knowing God will never leave us or forsake us? This is why spiritual maturity is unlike the physical maturing process. Our spiritual maturity becomes greater based on a deeper dependence on Him, rather than a deadening independence of Him. In other words, the tighter we hold His hand, the stronger and more peace-filled we become. One other distinction between spiritual maturity and real-life maturity is the area of our weaknesses. The world famously tells us not to admit weakness. When you do, you risk losing. Yet God says admitting weakness is the only way to win. The more we acknowledge how weak we are apart from Him, the more peace we have through Him. In 2 Corinthians 12:8–10, Paul talks about one of his weaknesses:

> Three times I pleaded with the Lord to take it away from me. But he said to me, "My grace is sufficient for you, for my power is made perfect in weakness." Therefore I will boast all the more gladly about my weaknesses, so that Christ's power may rest on me. That is why, for Christ's sake, I delight in weaknesses, in insults, in hardships, in persecutions, in difficulties. For when I am weak, then I am strong.

So going back to our Monopoly game, not only do we get out of jail by accepting Jesus, but we can constantly collect the proverbial $200 each time we "pass Go" and admit we need Him. The more we acknowledge our weaknesses, and choose to cling tighter to His hand, the more peace we'll have in our lives.

So we know we need Jesus to have peace. And we know we need to know how much we need Him to have more peace. It seems so simple. Yet most people will fight this for a lifetime, and sadly, some will even lose bankrupt.

This week will be an opportunity to have more peace in your life. Peace would not be something to get if we already knew we had it! This week you will look inside your personal peace bank. Don't be depressed if you're often overdrawn. Instead, look at your walks this week as hefty deposits.

This week, your Walk with Him program focuses on the promise of peace. Your challenge is to determine to walk in peace, no matter what else is going on in your life. You will walk a total of four times this week.

Walk with Him: Week Three Plan

Four walks: 45 minutes, 45 minutes, 30 minutes, 60 minutes

Week Three—Walk One—Day/Date: _____

45 minutes

Each walk this week will represent an area of our lives where we struggle to find peace. Next, you will pray for the peace of God to help handle your relationships, admit weakness, and ask for His strength.

Pre-Walk Challenge

You get to pick your friends, but God picks your family! This can be a lifetime struggle for many to accept. Even people who seem to have "perfect families," when you get to the nitty-gritty, still have plenty of dirt. Today your Walk with Him program is all about seeking peace within your home and with family members.

To have more peace in your life, you must seek peace with those placed in your life. Of course there are times when this seems impossible. Perhaps you have unresolved conflict with a loved one, and no matter what you've tried, they aren't interested in mending fences. Or if you approach them, they simply rehash old events for the sake of making their point for the three-hundredth time. It's okay to be in these situations. God goes through this with us regularly. Often He reaches out His hand to help, and we push it away.

To have peace within your home or family is up to you. Here's why: you get to control your words and your reactions. If you pursue peaceful conversations that overflow with sincere kindness, love, and mercy, the reception of them isn't yours to control. You can have immense peace within all of your family relationships if you've done everything within your power to pursue it. We may not always have perfect understanding of each other, but we can have peaceful exchanges with one another.

Before your walk, answer these questions:

What are the names of those living in your home?

_____

_____

What are the names of other family members who need prayer?

_____

_____

With whom do you need to pursue peace?

_____

_____

Go out for your 45-minute walk and think about some of your answers. As you head out, plan to go at a steady pace that you find challenging for the first 25 minutes. Turn around. Now make it your goal to get back in 20 minutes!

Post-Walk Chat

What are three things you can do to encourage and pursue peace with family members?

1. _____

_____

_____

2. _____

_____

_____

3. _____

_____

_____

Part of pursuing peace is letting go of the past. As you move forward this week, make it a regular prayer to see family members are people specifically chosen by God to be a part of your life.

Take the following verse and write it down somewhere you will see it:

Make every effort to live in peace with everyone and to be holy; without holiness no one will see the Lord. See to it that no one falls short of the grace of God and that

no bitter root grows up to cause trouble and defile many.
(Heb. 12:14–15)

Week Three—Walk Two—Day/Date: _____

45 minutes

Pre-Walk Challenge

Having peace-filled friendships is important. As Jesus's
disciples, we should aim each day at being more like Him.
The people we allow closest in our lives can either corrupt us
or create in us Christlike character. Please use today's walk to
pray for each of your friends. Also, use this time to ask God
for wisdom when it comes to whom you should invest more
time in. Also consider if you may need to distance yourself
from someone else.

Remember, there is a season for everything, including friendships. In fact, there are times when God may call us to spend
less time with someone we really enjoy being with, in order to
allocate time to reach out to someone else in need. Proverbs
27:17 says "As iron sharpens iron, so one person sharpens another." Think about the deeper meaning of this verse. When a
chef wants to make a dull knife cut better, he'll rub it against
his knife sharpener, which is basically another piece of metal.
As we rub up against our friends, they should be making us
better! Begin to use this verse as criteria for your friendships.
Seek to be a sharpener—and to become sharpened.

As you prepare for your physical walk, go ahead and break
down the time into three 15-minute segments. This will give
you a total of 45 minutes. Also, choose three friends by name,
and dedicate one segment to praying for each of them, and for
your friendship. It's not necessary for all three to be someone

you have spoken to recently. Perhaps there is someone you have unresolved conflict with, and it's about time you settle the dispute. During your Walk with Him workout, dedicate all of your friendships to the Lord and seek His blessing over each. For each segment of your walk, warm up for the first five minutes, pick up your speed to a steady, challenging pace for the next five minutes, and for the last five minutes gradually work up to a very intense walk. The goal for the last five minutes is to be nearly out of breath the entire time. Remember: you will do this 15-minute segment a total of three times!

Write down the names of the three friends you will pray for before you go:

1. _____

2. _____

3. _____

Post-Walk Chat

Welcome to the world of interval training. The purpose of today's walk was twofold. One was to focus on your friendships, and having peace about them and in them. The second was in relation to the intensity level of your workout.

In the last section of this book, we'll talk more about the importance of intensity. For now, I want you to recognize how it feels—and trust me, it's really good for you! For now, think of it like eating spinach as a kid. You may not have known exactly why you were doing it, but you believed your mom when she said it was good for you.

Answer the questions below about your walk today.

How do you feel physically?

_____

_____

What did your walk reveal to you today about your friendships?

_____

_____

Write down someone you could work to be a better friend to in the coming week.

_____

_____

Week Three—Walk Three—Day/Date: _____

30 minutes

Pre-Walk Challenge

We know peace is the opposite of war. Today's 30-minute walk is dedicated to national peace.

> I urge, then, first of all, that petitions, prayers, intercession and thanksgiving be made for all people—for kings and all those in authority, that we may live peaceful and quiet lives in all godliness and holiness. This is good, and pleases God our Savior, who wants all people to be saved and to come to a knowledge of the truth. (1 Tim. 2:1–4)

We need to be careful our *political* zeal doesn't get in the way of our *praying* zeal. Often we are quick to say how the country could best be run; however, who could argue it would be run the best if God were completely in control? Your walk today is a time for you to be thankful for living in a land of plenty, despite its imperfections. Commit to praying for peace in Washington and amongst our leaders, and for those making our laws. These verses in 1 Timothy tell us that praying for those in authority delivers peace.

Write the names of our current leaders in the spaces below. This will help you as you pray for each one. If you don't know their names, this is a great time to learn them!

President: _____

Vice President: _____

State Governor: _____

Speaker of the House: _____

Senate Majority and Minority Leaders: _____

_____

_____

Supreme Court Justices: _____

_____

_____

_____

_____

Keep your entire walk today at the same pace. On a scale of 1 to 10, try to maintain at least a level 7 in terms of intensity after the first 5 minutes and for the duration.

Post-Walk Chat

Praying for people you agree with is easy, but praying for people you may not agree with is tough! Peaceful living begins internally and in our quiet time. The bonus is the more we focus on things we control, such as how often we pray, whom we pray for, and what specifically we are praying about, the more likely we are to abandon the things we can't control (i.e., who currently holds an elected office). In other words, we can choose to shift our aggravation into an opportunity for spiritual growth with prayer.

What are your concerns about the current state of our government?

_____

_____

_____

_____

What are your specific prayers for our president?

_____

_____

_____

After this walk, consider sitting down with your family and talking with them about the importance of praying for those in authority.

Week Three—Walk Four—Day/Date: _____

60 minutes

Pre-Walk Challenge

So far, we've walked for more peace within our families, with our friends, and for our nation. Today we will walk for future peace. Actually, we'll focus on having more peace when it comes to the future. Most people get tripped up by fearing something that hasn't even happened yet. When it comes to losing weight, I've actually heard the argument, "Why bother? I always gain it back anyway."

There is no way to secure peace for the future if you are a person who allows today's troubles to control tomorrow's outcome. I recently did an internet search looking for stories on letting go of one's burdens. I ran across this great story.[2] Interestingly, the author is unknown. I picture the storyteller as a woman who subscribes to *Southern Living* and has a pretty nice life, but tends to sweat the small stuff. God wanted to use a simple carpenter to remind her about the true meaning of life. Sound familiar?

The carpenter I hired to help me restore an old farmhouse had just finished a rough first day on the job. A flat tire made him lose an hour of work, his electric saw quit, and now his ancient pickup truck refused to start. While I drove him home, he sat in stony silence.

On arriving, he invited me in to meet his family. As we walked toward the front door, he paused briefly at a small tree, touching the tips of the branches with both hands. When he opened the door, he underwent an amazing transformation. His tanned face wreathed in smiles, he hugged his two small children and gave his wife a kiss. Afterward he walked me to the car. We passed the tree and my curiosity got the better of me. I asked him about what I had seen him do earlier.

"Oh, that's my trouble tree," he replied. "I know I can't help having troubles on the job, but one thing for sure, troubles don't belong in the house with my wife and the children. So I just hang them on the tree every night when I come home. Then in the morning I pick them up again. Funny thing is," he smiled, "when I come out in the morning to pick 'em up, there ain't nearly as many as I remember hanging up the night before."

To me, this story is a beautiful reminder for us all. We can begin tomorrow with less worry if we will lay down today's worries, now.

The walk you are about to do will be your longest yet, an hour. As you work hard to become more fit, lose weight, and live well, remember peace and worry can't coexist. Take the time today to list some of your present worries and then make the decision to leave them on your walk. Just like the carpenter in the story, you may be surprised when it seems there are fewer worries when you return tomorrow!

Today's walk will be broken down into two parts.

Initially, warm up for 5 minutes. Now I know many people wonder, *What is a warm up?* Basically, it's the process of waking up your muscles and elevating your heart rate. For a walking warm up, don't think of it as a nice romantic stroll with your honey; instead, it's more like you're shopping and need to find a bathroom as soon as possible. You don't want to go so fast that it's obvious, but at the same time, you wouldn't consider stopping to try on a pair of shoes.

After your 5-minute warm up, spend the following 25 minutes walking with more intensity. Basically, you really need to find the bathroom and you could care less if everyone knows it, because the alternative won't be pretty! For the last 30 minutes, relax, but just a little. You're still not going to be trying on anything; however, you would quickly shuffle through some racks looking for your size, knowing the store is closing soon and the sale won't be on tomorrow.

As you begin to wrap up your walk, focus for the last few minutes on taking in deep breaths and breathing out all of today's worries. Here's a verse to remember on today's walk:

Therefore I tell you, do not worry about your life, what you will eat or drink; or about your body, what you will wear. Is not life more than food, and the body more than clothes? Look at the birds of the air; they do not sow or reap or store away in barns; yet your heavenly Father feeds them. Are you not much more valuable than they? (Matt. 6:24–26)

Post-Walk Chat

Obviously, "don't worry, be happy" was the theme for today's walk. But don't forget, it's because worry is a thief. Each and every time we spend a moment worrying, we have wasted a moment of having peace.

Pursing peace has been the crux of this week's Walk with Him program. But remember, you can't have peace with your family, friends, or anyone else if you don't have it within yourself. Part of maintaining a peaceful state of mind comes from protecting yourself from negative people and thoughts.

What is your definition of being at peace?

_____

_____

_____

Who are some people you know who seem to exemplify this?

_____

_____

In what ways could you protect your mind so you can have more peace?

_____

_____

_____

Can you agree that peace is something God can give us despite a weakened faith?

_____

_____

_____

Create a simple prayer for more peace in the space below:

_____

_____

_____

12

Walk with Him, Week Four

It's Time for More

*M*y mother has this catchphrase I heard countless times throughout my childhood: "Why bother doing something if you're not going to do it right?" As a teenager, I was quite sure this meant I should take a permanent break from my chores, like cleaning bathrooms. According to my mom, I often didn't seem to have a knack for doing it "right." Two things finally made me become better at it: allowance and trying to avoid restriction!

When it comes to walking with Him, you should work to get better for the same reasons. Seriously! The more you attempt while getting physically and spiritually fit, the more allowance you'll have. And if you aren't consistent, you may be grounded! Think of it like this: if you don't make regular efforts to become healthy and stay healthy, you'll have no strength or stamina to do the things you enjoy the most.

Now South Florida, where I live, is hot. Really, really hot! In fact, it's so hot we have a basketball team named the Heat! This past summer, we had a record seventy-nine days straight where the temperature hit over 90 degrees.[3]

It seemed so unbearable. Honestly, I wanted to see about getting a water-resistant laptop. I thought working in the swimming pool might be a helpful way to handle the insane heat. But it also made me realize heat can be a good thing. It made me appreciate air-conditioning, cold water, and frozen yogurt.

Now that you've got the discipline of walking down, three weeks into the program, it's time to stop seeing exercise as uncomfortable and instead see its benefits. Up until this point, I have purposely not put an emphasis on nutrition or kept close tabs on your intensity. All this is going to change this week. You see, I know you can't be competitive without consistency, even if we're only talking about competing with yourself. This is why the first three weeks I focused more on simply getting you to show up, and teaching you to utilize the greatest trainer of all time—God. However, it's time to turn up the thermostat! Or, as we Florida basketball fans say when the season commences, the Heat is on!

As we are about to kick it into high gear, you'll need to know why it's important to learn to walk stronger and better.

The Pay for Performance Advantage

Now, I have been a salesperson most of my life. In the past, I have sold advertising for magazines, jewelry, purses, and a few other more embarrassing things. (Okay, it was cheesecakes—before my weight loss, of course!) I really like the concept of paying anyone and everyone based on his or her performance. To me, this means the harder people work, the more they can be rewarded. When I hired our first babysitter several years ago, I tried to get her to see my point. Here was my offer: a dollar if the kids are sleeping when we get home. A dollar for doing all the dishes. A dollar if the children have no cuts or bruises. And a dollar if the house isn't burned down. For some reason, this didn't fly!

Nearly everyone likes the comfort of being paid a set salary without the pressure of having to perform. However, when it comes to exercise, know this: it's all pay for performance! Sure, there is a small guarantee. For example, if you show up and do the bare minimum, you will burn some calories and feel a little better. However, the more consistent you are, and the greater intensity you put forth, the more the return!

Restriction Is No Fun!

Here's a thought: How much time would you have to do fun stuff if you're always busy doing not-so-fun stuff? Obviously, none!

I'm amazed when I meet someone who tells me they have too many health issues to exercise. Often they will have a crazy schedule that includes taking medications, seeing doctors, and so on. Imagine how much time they'd free up if they used more energy to exercise instead of focusing their energy on their health problems. Most health issues can be improved with proper nutrition and regular movement.

Have you tried to use the scotch tape and you find the end is lost somewhere on the spool? It can be totally annoying. Plus you can waste lots of time trying to figure out where the tape starts. The problem is you can't use any of the tape until you solve the real issue. Hopefully by now in your Walk

119

with Him program you have done well and put in the time learning to be consistent. Essentially, you've found the starting point. Now it's time to do some fixing—or use the "tape," so to speak—and this is going to happen as we begin to flavor your fitness program with intensity! Remember, you can't get better at something until you are doing it in the first place. This fourth week of your program, we will spice it up and turn up the heat!

Don't be afraid. We won't do anything too crazy! Really, I'm serious. Weight-loss reality shows drive me nuts! Usually you see a television trainer attempt to make someone go from being a nonexerciser to an avid fitness buff (who works out six hours a day), in just a matter of weeks! And I'll admit, it can be really exciting to watch. But think about it. These folks on television are trying to prove themselves worthy as they share their tear-filled stories of rejection and self-loathing. And it's designed for our entertainment. The truth is, no one would tune in to *The Slowest Loser*!

Ask yourself this: Why would a radical and rapid approach to solving a lifelong struggle stick when the pressure to perform is gone? We know, by seeing those famous "where are they now" stories, they don't. This is not how real life works. Time and tests are what reassure us we are capable of staying on track. Think about it. Do you want a doctor to operate on you who just finished an internet speed course on "How to Do Surgery"? Not me. I want the guy who went to school for many years and has already done countless operations. This way I know he has put in the required time to be able to do a top-notch job. If you will continue to be consistent, occasionally adding competition will be more like icing on the cake.

When my littlest son, Luke, was learning to read, he started with small books that had five or ten words on a page. Next, he graduated to mini-chapter books. Eventually, he went on to longer books with bigger words. I'll never forget him ambitiously begging me to buy him a book at Barnes and Noble that was out of his league. Not only did it have too many pages, it also had lots of words I knew he couldn't comprehend.

Well I, of course, got the book. How could I say no to his desire to overachieve? Especially because I knew exactly where he got this trait from. Within one hour he had thrown the book across the living room. My little genius was mad and frustrated. It wasn't that he was a poor reader, it was that he was trying to do something well he hadn't learned yet.

Today, he reads a full three grades higher than the one he's in, and it's not because after the book-throwing incident I said, "From now on we'll read only books that are way too hard for you." Instead, it was because he went back to reading books he was ready for, and worked his way up from there.

It is my heart's desire for you to want to walk strong and live well for many years to come. Now it's time to begin focusing on adding a greater challenge. This is when you will begin to feel stronger while you're walking. Don't forget: seeing regular improvement will help you always be on the lookout for it! This week you'll walk a total of five times. The first two walks will be somewhat challenging, the third will be a recovery or restful walk, and the last two walks will be the most intense.

Again, we will walk for a specific length of time as we have in the past three weeks; however, you will also now walk to become faster. I understand you may not be ready to invest in a gadget such as a GPS to measure your precise pace, or a heart-rate monitor. However, I will get into the benefits of both of these in a later chapter.

For now, I'm going to teach you two simple ways to measure your intensity that will serve as guidelines on your walks this week. Take the time to become familiar with them. I will ask you to use them on all five walks:

1. The Pledge Test
2. Perceived Rate of Exertion (We'll call it your PRE)

In addition, each walk has a catchphrase or a tagline to go along with it. In each pre-walk challenge you will learn more about how to integrate this phrase into your walk. Be ready when you return to reflect for a few minutes on the thrill that comes with knowing you're making headway!

The Pledge Test

The Pledge test is based on (yes, you likely guessed it) the Pledge of Allegiance! When it comes to exercise, talking while you're moving is one of the simplest ways you can measure your intensity. Know this: other than the first few minutes you'll spend warming up, you should not be able to carry on a conversation effortlessly, as if you were strolling down the street on a cool, crisp, autumn day, window shopping with a girlfriend. However, on the other extreme, you also shouldn't be gasping for air while you walk, to the point that an exercise partner would wonder if she should go get help!

The best-case scenario is for you to know how to gauge your intensity alone. (Having a walking partner isn't and shouldn't always be an option.) While having a conversation with yourself to check your breathing is fine by me, you may want to avoid getting carried off to the funny farm! This is why the Pledge test works. It is something you can do quickly, easily, and many times throughout a walk. It will also help you gauge your cardiovascular improvement.

Here is the Pledge of Allegiance broken down into four lines:

(Line 1) I pledge allegiance to the flag of the United States of America

(Line 2) And to the republic for which it stands

(Line 3) One nation, under God, indivisible

(Line 4) With liberty and justice for all

During your walk, periodically take the Pledge test. Be careful not to place your right hand over your heart. Someone driving by may think you're having a heart attack and call 9-1-1!

Here's how each line corresponds with your four training zones: warm-up, endurance, strength, and athletic.

Warm-up zone: You can say all four lines, or most of it, with just one breath.

Endurance zone: You can still make it through most, if not all, of the third line before needing another breath.

Strength zone: You need to take a breath somewhere in the second line.

Athletic zone: You need to stop and take a breath anywhere in the first line.

Your PRE—Perceived Rate of Exertion

Your PRE is basically a number you determine and use to evaluate your level of intensity during an exercise session.

The scale goes from 1–10; 1 being the easiest and 10 being the most challenging:

1–3 You are feeling good, and you think exercise is awesome!

4–5 You are beginning to watch the clock.

6–7 You wonder if this was a bad idea.

8 You just want the birds to stop singing!

9 You might throw up.

10 "This doesn't look like Kansas anymore."

I'm sure you get the idea. Levels 1–3 are when you can breathe comfortably, and have just started out. Levels 4–5 are the endurance zone. Somewhere in this rate of breathing is where a marathon is run. Levels 6–7 are where exercise is both mental and physical. Here is where you really start hoping it won't be long until you're done. This is also the line between the endurance zone and the strength zone.

Level 8 is when you are working out hard enough that you need to focus. I joked about the birds, but basically it's when you need to concentrate. This is a full-on strength zone, bordering on athletic zone conditioning. Once you hit level 9, you know it won't be long until you need to stop. Liken this to someone going for a sprint. The goal is to push the limits of the cardiovascular system.

Most people will never get to level 10. Level 10 is best done under the advisement of a doctor and is often referred to as a stress test. There is no good reason for you to try to go to a 10 on your own, anyway.

Walk with Him: Week Four Plan

Five walks: 45 minutes, 45 minutes, 20 minutes, 45 minutes, 30 minutes

Week Four—Walk One—Day/Date: _____

45 minutes

Pre-Walk Challenge

"IT'S YOUR BIRTHDAY!"

I don't gamble, but I'd be willing to make a small wager it's not your real birthday. However, if it is, and you have this walk planned for today, that is beyond cool! But any given day can really feel like your birthday, if you want it to.

Now, my husband and I have entirely different views on the importance of a birthday. In his mind, it's just another day. In my mind, it's a national event to be celebrated by all for a solid week. I actually think employers should automatically give a week's paid vacation to each employee on their birthday week so they enjoy it in every way! Why not seriously celebrate the fact you were born? I always sign my name with my life verse, Psalm 139:13–16:

> For You formed my inward parts;
> > You covered me in my mother's womb.
> I will praise You, for I am fearfully and wonderfully
> > made;
> > Marvelous are Your works,
> > And that my soul knows very well.
> My frame was not hidden from You,
> > When I was made in secret,
> > And skillfully wrought in the lowest parts of the
> > earth.
> Your eyes saw my substance, being yet unformed.
> > And in Your book they all were written,
> > The days fashioned for me,
> > When as yet there were none of them. (NKJV)

Here's why I love these verses: they are full of promise when it comes to who I am and why I'm here. God is saying we are entirely His design, every part of us!

Repeat this: "I am celebrating my life today! I am thankful I have been wonderfully and fearfully made. I will no longer

125

complain about parts of me that I can't change. Praise God He has a unique plan for each day of my life."

Your walk is for 45 minutes. I want you to use the Pledge test several times today. Begin with a 5-minute warm up. Next, focus on your breathing, and every 5 minutes work toward walking fast enough that you must take a breath by the end of the first line of the Pledge. After you hit this level of intensity several times, spend 5 minutes walking at a pace where you can get through the first three lines before needing a breath. Do this until your time is up.

Post-Walk Chat

Well . . . how do you feel?

_____

_____

_____

_____

In what ways did the Pledge test help you?

_____

_____

_____

Since I told you it's your birthday, how did you approach your walk differently?

_____

_____

Week Four—Walk Two—Day/Date: _____

45 minutes

Pre-Walk Challenge

"LOVE IS IN THE AIR!"

Nothing is cuter to me than watching my children react to seeing Keith and I steal a kiss. Our sixteen-year-old, Ashley, might say something like, "Really, Mom . . . really, Dad?" Our next in line, Kayla, who also happens to be a little sassy, might mutter, "Isn't that why you share a bedroom?" Jake would have one word: "Disgusting." And little Luke would say, "Daddy, leave my mommy alone!" . . . but likely Keith and I would laugh, ignore them, and smooch again!

Today's catchphrase is "Love is in the air." I'm not talking exclusively about romantic love. I mean in terms of trying to find ways to outwardly display love to those closest to you in your life. We've all been guilty of assuming someone knows we love them even though we make little effort to show them. On today's walk, you will dedicate a few minutes to thinking of a few ways to show love to those God has placed in your life. It can be as simple as cleaning out your sister's car, or baking your kids some banana bread. And a little love note goes a long way!

Today's walk is also 45 minutes. You will be using your PRE (perceived rate of exertion) for today's walk. The goal for your first 15 minutes is to go from level 1 to level 7 and then back to level 6. The next 15 minutes, you will go from level 6 to level 9. And for the last 15 minutes, you will go down to level 3 and then work your way up to level 8, and finish by going all the way back down to level 1.

Post-Walk Chat

"LOVE IS IN THE AIR!"

Today's walk was all about love. Take a look at the description of love from 1 Corinthians 13:

> Love is patient, love is kind. It does not envy, it does not boast, it is not proud. It does not dishonor others, it is not self-seeking, it is not easily angered, it keeps no record of wrongs. Love does not delight in evil but rejoices with the truth. It always protects, always trusts, always hopes, always perseveres. Love never fails. (vv. 4–8)

This is a charge for us when it comes to how we show love.

Who will you try to show more love to today?

_____

_____

Any ideas on how?

_____

_____

If love never fails, and we know God loves us, then shouldn't we succeed at everything God is helping us to accomplish? What are your thoughts?

_____

_____

By the end of this walk, you should have a better understanding of your perceived exertion. Explain how your workout changed as you used the Pledge test and the PRE test. For example: Did you work harder? Or did you pace yourself better?

_____

_____

_____

Week Four—Walk Three—Day/Date: _____

20 minutes

Pre-Walk Challenge

"BEAUTY IS IN THE EYE OF THE BEHOLDER."

Each one of us has been rigged to see beauty differently. Do you know that in some cultures, being overweight is considered an attractive quality? In fact, when food was scarce and hunting was the primary source of income, having a heavy wife was proof you were successful. Much like you or I owning a mansion or driving a Ferrari.

Seeking to be more beautiful is exhausting if you let others define it for you. True beauty is unfading.

Go out for your easy 20-minute walk today. Use the Pledge test and the PRE test. In terms of the Pledge, be sure to be able to say nearly the entire thing in one breath for the entire walk. When using the PRE test, stay between levels 3 and 6 the entire time. Also, be thinking about your definition of true beauty.

Post-Walk Chat

True beauty to me is:

_____

_____

Ways I can feel more beautiful by my definition above:

_____

_____

_____

Proverbs 31:30

> Charm is deceptive, and beauty is fleeting; but a woman who fears the LORD is to be praised.

Week Four—Walk Four—Day/Date: _____

45 minutes

Pre-Walk Challenge

"THE HILLS ARE ALIVE."

The lyrics "The hills are alive" are from *The Sound of Music*. It's hard to forget actress Julie Andrews singing this tune with her arms swinging freely in the air. It is a reminder of carefree living, and feeling great while looking at simple things. Your walk today is meant to be simple and special.

Where I live, there are virtually no hills. For me to feel like I am walking uphill I either need to use a treadmill or take deep strides while I move my legs and arms rapidly. The concept for today's Walk with Him is to have you focus on simulating hills through your walk intensity. If you happen to live in an area where there are actual hills available, great. You'll want to use them as part of your route.

During this 45-minute walk, plan on going to the top of ten hills during your workout. Take the Pledge test on your walk, and be sure to get to the point where you must take a breath somewhere in the first line at least ten times. Go out and feel alive!

Post-Walk Chat

So the hills are alive, but do you feel dead?

_____

_____

At what point in the 45 minutes did you feel the most challenged?

_____

_____

_____

Where did you see beauty in something simple?

_____

_____

_____

Week Four—Walk Five—Day/Date: _____

30 minutes

Pre-Walk Challenge

"Stayin' alive."

Having parents who love to throw big karaoke parties has caused me to be a bit of a disco fan. The music of the '70s just screams, "Let's party!" I know the past several weeks have literally had lots of ups and downs. But I hope you are encouraged today. You are more alive than ever before. And here's the best news: you now have a solid plan to stay feeling this way!

Today's 30-minute walk will be the most challenging yet. I want you to focus on the workout today in terms of a bigger picture than simply getting it over with. Instead, set out on your walk today with the fierceness of a person who is determined to live the rest of her life strong and fit. However, don't forget: becoming better at anything requires regular training. Even world-renowned surgeons will take refresher courses or seminars to learn something new. As you walk strong for 30 minutes today, use the PRE test as your guide. After a 5-minute warm up, keep your number of perceived exertion between levels 7 and 9 the entire time.

Take this verse for motivation!

> Don't you realize that in a race everyone runs, but only one person gets the prize? So run to win! (1 Cor. 9:24 NLT)

Post-Walk Chat

I have entered many races already knowing there was no way I would win. But the key is not to run or walk with this mentality. The prize we are walking for is subjective. Each one of us considers a win to be something different. Some people need to lose 50 pounds, so losing weight is the victory. Some just need to get off medication and feel better. They are looking to win back their health.

What are you trying to win with your Walk with Him program?

_____

_____

Do you think you are getting closer to winning than you were four weeks ago? In what ways?

_____

_____

_____

What day was your favorite walk over the past four weeks?

_____

_____

_____

Why?

_____

_____

_____

Where do you go from here?

_____

_____

_____

Part 3

The Weight

13

Need and Want
Aren't the Same

I'm finally going to bring "it" up. Yes, it's a "weighty subject," but it must be addressed. It's time for me to give you some straight talk when it comes to shedding pounds. Now I know you may be thinking, *Chantel, if I just walk a lot more, surely the weight will eventually just melt off, right?*

Believe me, I'd love to say yes. But reality forbids me. You see, dealing with my weight has been a lifelong battle for me. Exercise has proven to be a key management tool, but certainly not a cure-all. Therefore, in this chapter, I'm going to share with you some things I've never said before regarding real, long-term weight loss. Just remember: I've been on this journey for over ten years now. I've learned the only way to stay this course is to always look ahead. In fact, looking back will do nothing more than cause a crick in your neck. I am convinced today, more than ever, that for any self-improvement attempt to stick there needs to be room for new discovery.

Have you ever powered up your computer and seen the message flash on the screen, "your updates are now ready"? I've learned the hard way what happens if you keep ignoring this friendly reminder. Eventually you'll run into a problem. Often your computer will slow down or stop working altogether. What I'm trying to say is this: don't be surprised if I update something in this book regarding my views on the process of weight loss and the reasons for it. I simply want to help you continue your journey, fix glitches, or help make you aware of potential problems.

Here's the real deal about how to lose weight and keep it off, for life! Repeat after me: "Stepping on a scale constantly is silly." I'm totally serious! Hear me out. I'm not saying all scales are unnecessary. There are times when you should weigh yourself regularly and precision is critical. For example, if you are one of the many folks practicing to become a professional boxer, monitoring your weight closely to stay within a particular weight class is very important. Also, if you are an astronaut who is waiting on a list to be called upon any day to take a trip to space, keeping track of your exact weight is vital. However, when it comes to long-term weight management, hopping on and off a scale constantly is definitely a bad idea.

In fact, I will go as far as to say if you are getting on a scale a few times a day, you may as well be hopping on and off a roller-coaster ride at the county fair. The problem is you'll begin to see yourself as if you are looking in one of those distorted mirrors in the funhouse. But it won't be funny. Eventually you'll end up allowing a piece of metal to deliver joy or steal your sanity!

The truth is that ten out of ten people die. In fact, it's the one statistic that really doesn't need a reference. I've never heard someone whisper at a funeral, "Wow, how much do you think she weighs?" Once you're gone, you're gone, right? And how many pounds you weigh at the time is pretty much irrelevant. Yet I can't imagine how much time we, as a society, will waste obsessing about this number as if it's going to be embroidered on our uniforms in heaven.

Since I am a native Floridian, Disney World is a frequent vacation destination. When we arrive at the Magic Kingdom, first, we pay to park. Next we are directed to a parking lot. Then we pay again to enter "the park." Once we've settled up, a big decision needs to be made: What means of transportation will we take to get to the other side, where the Magic Kingdom awaits? There are two choices, a monorail or a ferry boat.

I can remember my parents handling this dilemma back when I was a little girl taking this same trip to Disney. Most often, they'd make us wait in the long line to take one of the ferry boats. They said the ride was more enjoyable. We kids argued, but they promised it would be worth the wait. To me, the ride always seemed like it took forever. As we'd set out, the castle was faint in the distance. As the boat chugged along, little by little, it would begin to get closer and closer. And after saying to my mom at least a hundred times, "I just can't wait," we would finally arrive. I'll never forget the sights and sounds . . . popcorn, music, smiling faces—this place seemed truly magical!

Flash-forward thirty years, and I'm now taking my kids. Now, I'll be honest, these days my gang wants to take the monorail. Here's why: It's much, much faster. And because Keith and I have been there many times, we know the hassle factor of the process of getting to the other side quite well. This means we don't even try to persuade them into taking the boat. In our minds, we must hurry up and get on the monorail so we can *get there*. We wouldn't want to waste a minute.

And it never fails. Within the first few minutes of arriving, we all look confusedly at each other as we try to figure out where we should go. And why? Well, it's because we got there so fast we forgot to talk about it and figure it out ahead of time. Did I forget to mention this is supposed to be a vacation, like an enjoyable retreat from real life? Yet on many trips the past few years, I've felt like I may as well be running late trying to catch the subway so I can ring the opening bell on Wall Street. Something is not right about this picture!

I figured it out. And it has little to do with being a grown-up now, with less patience and a more realistic perception. The problem isn't how I see Disney; instead, it's how my children see it. And it's not remotely the same. And that is because the anticipation factor of arriving gets lost in the hurried hustle to "get there." You see, it's so fast, something valuable is forgotten: where we're actually going! So when we finally do get there, the kids don't fully appreciate where we have gotten to.

When it comes to losing weight, I've taken the monorail many, many times, and I finally took the ferry boat. Here's the difference. The monorail of dieting can be quite efficient. There are lots of ways one can lose weight, fast! But chances are, the lack of a reasonable number of calories will turn into obsession as you try to justify the whole process by hitting a magical number on the scale as quickly as possible. Sadly, once you've arrived, you won't have a clue what to do next. But as long as it includes eating, you're in!

Wanting things quickly is a universal problem. Who enjoys watching television in real time? Especially now that fast-forwarding through commercials is an option. Yet who do you think pays for the television show? Its advertisers do. These days actors must overexaggerate their love for dish soap in a totally unrelated scene so they can still collect a big paycheck.

If you want to lose weight fast, have at it! But know this: at some point, a challenging situation will arise, and because you haven't invested time working hard and anticipating success, you'll need to become crafty in order to still maintain your weight loss. I'm not saying this can't be done, but I certainly know what you're getting into if you're in a hurry.

In addition, when someone attempts to lose weight so they can see the scale smile back at them daily, or even hourly, a love/hate relationship with food often ignites. When they eat much less and see the number go down, avoiding food is rewarding. Then when they give in and eat something meant to be delicious, and the number goes up, food becomes an enemy. It drives me crazy to hear someone say, "I cheated this past weekend." And they next confess they ate chocolate chip cookies, a few of which never even made it into the oven.

Here I was ready to take them to a marriage counselor, and all they meant was they indulged in something sweet. Don't hear me wrong. Eating way too many chocolate chip cookies can certainly be considered gluttony, but is it cheating? I looked up a definition of cheating. It was quite interesting: "a deliberate dishonest transaction." It's no wonder so many people feel like they are in prison when it comes to their relationship with food. On the other hand, because many people, including myself, have been or are in a love affair with chocolate chip cookies, I must address the need for weight loss. For many reasons, losing weight can be life saving. Maintaining a healthy weight delivers the following:

Fewer joint and muscle pains
Greater ability to join in desired activities
Better regulation of bodily fluids and blood pressure
Reduced burden on your heart and circulatory system
Better sleep patterns
More effective metabolism of sugars and carbohydrates
Reduced risk for heart disease and certain cancers

Most importantly, and you'll never hear this on a weight-loss reality series, remaining overweight has the potential to shorten your ability to serve God and fulfill His unique purpose for your life. Know this: being overweight and being weight-obsessed can take identical tolls. Trust me, I've been on this slippery slope.

In order to avoid going down that slope, or to recognize if you already are, you'll need to determine whether you *need* to lose weight or if you *want* to lose weight. There is a difference. For those who need to lose weight, there is a potential health hazard involved. Being overweight is infringing on their ability to embrace life fully. For those who want to lose weight, it's perhaps a little more about vanity. I'm not saying this is always a bad thing, as long as it's kept in check.

I'm going to give you some simple guidelines to help you figure out where you're at. I realize everyone's body is different. Therefore, it's possible to seem to be on the cusp of being overweight, in terms of Body Mass Index (BMI), but in reality your body is healthy. This can happen to people whose muscle mass weighs more than that of most other folks. Perhaps they are extremely athletic. Since muscle weighs more than fat, this higher weight will deliver a higher BMI. However, the person's waist circumference will paint a truer picture of their fitness.

One more thing: while having an accurate body fat test would be optimal, it's not necessary. I'm not trying to set a gold standard here to tell you it's time to lose weight. Instead, I want to equip you with solid information so you can paint your own picture and decide for yourself. In addition, I feel it's beneficial for you to know if your expressed desire to lose weight is based on want or need—or simply an inaccurate self-perception.

First, measure your waist circumference—this is basically the narrowest part of your abdomen. If you have a difficult time finding it, you can also measure about an inch above your belly button.

I realize this seems too simple. However, the amount of fat stored around your midsection is critical in determining if your weight is causing a potential health risk. According to the National Heart, Lung, and Blood Institute, a woman with a waist circumference over 35 inches or a man with a waist circumference over 40 inches is at a higher risk for stroke, heart attack, and type two diabetes.[4]

Next, calculate your Body Mass Index.

You BMI is a number calculated based on your height and weight. This is a far better way to determine if your weight falls in a healthy range than using a scale alone. Remember, the number on the scale is a combination of muscle, fat, and water, which is guaranteed to cause regular fluctuation. Just ask any woman who weighs herself before beginning her menstrual cycle. However, adding in your height helps to personalize the number.

How to Calculate Your BMI

Take your weight in pounds, multiply it by 703, then divide that number by your height in inches. Take this number and divide it by your height in inches again. This final number is your BMI.

Your weight _____ ×703 ÷ your height (in inches) _____ = _____ ÷ your height again (in inches) = _____. This is your BMI.

The BMI chart is as follows:

BMI below 18.5 = Underweight

BMI 18.5–24.9 = Normal

BMI 25.0–29.9 = Overweight

BMI 30.0 and above = Obese

To determine desirable body weight without factoring in your BMI, try this simple method as described below:

1. Women: 100 pounds of body weight for the first 5 feet of height, 5 pounds for each additional inch.
2. Men: 106 pounds of body weight for the first 5 feet of height, 6 pounds for each additional inch.

Add 10 percent for a large frame size, and subtract 10 percent for a small frame size.

Determine Frame Size

To determine body frame size, measure the wrist with a tape measure and use the following chart to determine whether the person has a small, medium, or large frame.

WOMEN: under 5'2"

Small frame = wrist size less than 5.5"

Medium frame = wrist size 5.5"–5.75"
Large frame = wrist size over 5.75"

WOMEN: 5'2"–5'5"
Small frame = wrist size less than 6.0"
Medium frame = wrist size 6.0"–6.25"
Large frame = wrist size over 6.25"

WOMEN: over 5'5"
Small frame = wrist size less than 6.25"
Medium frame = wrist size 6.25"–6.5"
Large frame = wrist size over 6.5"

MEN: over 5'5"
Small frame = wrist size 5.5"–6.5"
Medium frame = wrist size 6.5"–7.5"
Large frame = wrist size over 7.5"

Now that we've talked about the real deal when it comes to why we might need or want to lose weight, it's now time to get into the fun part—how! Just remember, you're incorporating all of this into your Walk with Him program. This means you should use your walking time to remember why you don't want to miss the boat.

14

You May Just Stink at Math!

I can't begin to count the number of emails I've received from men and women asking me to tell them how to address a loved one concerning their weight problem. In the past, I've told them what I've found out to be true myself: don't bother preaching in your own backyard!

Here's why: people we love want to know we love them for what's on the inside. Therefore, if we attempt to talk to them about their weight, often what they hear is we're having trouble loving them because of their appearance. This is especially true when it comes to women and teenage girls. While this may be the last thing we want to say, it doesn't change what our loved one will likely feel if we try.

Remember, when you say something of a sensitive nature to someone, it's not just a matter of perfect timing or proper wording. The reception lies within the other person's ability to hear. For example, if you have an uncle who has a drinking problem and you tell him it's time to stop, chances are he won't listen, especially because he's just gotten in a fight with his wife and she called him a drunk. Likely, after your attempt to chat, he'll storm off to the local bar.

The same principle applies to a person with a weight problem. They are often dealing with an internal fight that never seems to let up. Don't forget, every mirror is a smack in their face. If you try to approach them, you may actually be adding more fuel to the fire of despair that is already burning inside their mind and heart. But this doesn't mean it can't be done. In addition, if you are in need of shedding some pounds yourself, I want to give you a fresh change of perspective.

I once sat across from a woman who was at least 100 pounds overweight and said the words, "You really don't have a weight issue." She looked at me as if I were insane. I was prepared to defend my statement. It broke my heart to hear her go on and on about how fat she was, how she hated herself, and what a terrible person she had become. I knew an emotion-filled "but you're so beautiful" response from me was the last thing she needed. Not because she may have thought I was trying only to pacify her, but because her real, root problem was the belief she was too far gone. She simply needed to see her failure as something solvable.

"Sister, you have a math problem, not a weight issue!" I said. She looked baffled, and then she laughed in a confused sort of way. I went on a little further. "To lose weight, just recognize you just stink at math! That is math, in terms of the calories you've been taking in through eating and then not using up."

By using this approach, I was trying to help her subtract emotion and self-pity from the equation. I knew if she'd simplify her problem, she'd begin to see a solution might be within her reach. The next step, I told her, was to begin doing her homework. In other words, she needed to exercise more and research healthy eating. Finally, I told her if she kept showing up for class (in other words, do what she needed to each day to cut calories), her math skills would sharpen. Eventually her body would reflect this, and she'd begin to look and feel amazing!

I also reminded her that not everyone is rigged to be a math whiz. Therefore, she didn't need to stress out about trying to get to an unrealistic size. Instead, she should concentrate on just getting better, one day at a time. Eventually she might make the honor roll, or in this case, go to the next level of fitness or get into a smaller pair of jeans. Or she might just end up with a high C—instead of the F she currently had. Her response was awesome! It was as if I totally took all the pressure off her to lose lots of weight, and instead offered her hope that she could begin to see consistent improvement. Ask yourself: would it be better to have a high C than an F? Of course! If everyone could begin to believe this when it comes to tackling weight loss, there would be a lot fewer people in our society failing at the math of weight maintenance.

Frankly, I don't care what "study" reports that millions of folks are special enough to defy math and therefore need radical weight loss surgery because they are physically incapable of losing weight. As a woman who was once a prime candidate and who now spends lots of time helping obese people, I can swallow the pill that some individuals have a much greater challenge losing weight than others. The truth is, in most cases a person willing to undergo radical surgery is simply a person who is frustrated and looking for a forced means of becoming disciplined.

I was recently in an assisted living facility for seniors, and as I took a good look around, I noticed many different shapes and sizes. Now remember, these folks all have closely monitored diets. They also don't drive. This means they don't have access to fast-food or big bags of potato chips, either. Yet, by the looks of everyone, no one was malnourished. You would think they'd all be scrawny and wasting away. But most of them seemed to be maintaining a pretty healthy body weight. In fact, I was ready to glue many of them to a walker instead of seeing them just sitting around.

My experience and research over the years regarding metabolism reminded me why this was the case. Our bodies are constantly trying to adapt and accommodate the calories we regularly take in and then burn off. Most of these elderly people maintained the weight they were at when their level of activity began to reduce drastically and their calorie intake became consistent. The only way someone in this situation would lose weight would be by experiencing a major calorie deprivation or by having a significant increase in activity. You and I are the same as these senior citizens. You see, our bodies are rigged for efficiency. Therefore, weight gain is really the by-product of an efficient machine, your body, trying to create a reserve in case there is a future complication in getting fuel or burning it!

Back when I first began to truly understand this whole process, I felt liberated. With all my previous diet attempts I was so focused on working a system, I never understood "the system." Think about it this way: my husband is a trim carpenter. Do you think he would pay another man to put up crown molding in our home? I can tell you without any hesitation, no way! Why? Because it's something he knows how to do. And even if he doesn't feel like doing it, he'd still have trouble paying someone else, because he is perfectly qualified and has worked hard to master the skill. One of my greatest prayers for anyone who has been stuck in the whole diet drama is for them to become calorie experts and possess a clear comprehension of how their body stores and burns calories. This will eliminate their need to look any further than God's help to work the system He designed—because they are qualified, and have mastered the skills they need. They don't need anyone else—or any fancy diet—to do it for them.

Once you "get it," reality sets in. There really are no short cuts. Sure, there are things you can do to lose weight really fast, such as a dramatic cut in calories along with a crazy amount of exercise. However, at some point you won't be able to keep this up. Then you'll have a problem. Remember in school when your math teacher said "Be sure to show me all the work"? This was because she wanted to make sure you understood how to solve the problem. If all she saw was a correct answer, she'd think you took a short-cut. While the right answer was still right at the time, a good teacher would want to make sure you understood how to solve the problem every time you had to solve another one like it.

When it comes to dealing with the calories in and calories out system, learn to do the math correctly, even if it is the long way. My daughter is studying pre-calculus at the moment, and a small part of me thinks it's a waste. I never use this kind of math in real life. But we must realize the math of how our bodies store and use food is something we will be able to use for the rest of our lives.

I'm going to call it like it is. Most of us at some point chose to sit in the corner with our arms crossed, refusing to do the work to lose weight, unwilling to sit down, grab a pencil, and go for it. Maybe it's because we forget to raise our hands for help, literally, or maybe it's because calorie deprivation sounds depressing. And it can be. Any sort of deprivation is not going to be a Sunday picnic complete with fried chicken, mac-n-cheese, watermelon, and potato salad. But deprivation doesn't need to be depressing if you will begin to understand how to bring a little of the picnic into your life each day. For example, watermelon is awesome. And a piece of fried chicken on occasion is also okay. It's just you can't have all of it all the time.

I'm going to teach you how to eat foods that will ignite and fuel your metabolism. Next, it will be up to you to do the math. Don't forget, as you also subtract the calories you'll be burning with your Walk with Him program, you'll eventually be an expert mathematician yourself.

So now, pull up a chair. I'm going to bring in some additional expert help. Elisa Zied is a registered dietician and the author of several great books on healthy eating.[5] In addition, she has become a personal friend. I refer to her because I know she has a unique passion to give solid scientific information. She has also been a spokesperson for the American Dietetic Association as well as a regular contributor on MSNBC.

According to Elisa, these are the approximate calorie needs of women, not taking into account exercise that's in addition to just "doing life."

WOMEN

Age	Calories
19–25	About 2,000
26–50	About 1,800
51 and above	About 1,600

Note: the reason calorie needs decrease is to compensate for a natural decrease in metabolism due to the muscle loss that comes along with the beauty of age. Wouldn't you think that if we must deal with wrinkles, a little more chocolate would be okay? And it is okay . . . but you must exercise for it and strength train to maintain muscle.

MEN

Age	Calories
21–40	About 2,400
41–60	About 2,200
61 and above	About 2,000

So, now that you have some numbers, next let's talk about what they really mean.

A pound of body weight equals 3,500 calories of energy. Calories are energy. If you took your body weight and multiplied it times 3,500, this is how much energy you have in the bank. Now, this doesn't mean a 200-pound person has 700,000 calories available to go out and run 700 miles without consuming food. Not every part of your body weight can be broken down into energy. Take two people who both weigh 200 pounds and are both stranded on a raft in the middle of the ocean without food. One is a woman with 45 percent body fat, and the other is a man with 7 percent body fat. Speaking exclusively on a physical level, the woman has a much better chance of surviving longer. Now, this is not to suggest everyone needs to maintain a high amount of body fat just in case the cruise ship sinks. In fact, it's the opposite. If you have an unhealthy excess of body fat, which can be determined by a high BMI as discussed in the last chapter, you must force your body into survival mode so it will use some of that extra fat for energy—but how?

It's the math. You must burn more calories than your body is taking in. Notice the key word: YOU! It's your body and your metabolism. Therefore, the rate at which you burn what you burn is likely not the same as Betty-Jo who lives next door and weighs 102 pounds dripping wet. Also, Betty-Jo may have a personal trainer and run fifty miles a week . . .

In the past, for weight loss, I have recommended most women keep their calories at around 1,500 a day and men at about 1,800. This is to go along with five days a week of exercise that averages 45 minutes each session. I still feel this is a realistic number that works to fit high-quality foods into your daily diet that will be satisfying and still not compromise nutrients. Any weight loss plan that recommends a calorie intake less than this may put your overall health in danger. This includes your organ function and bone density.

As you begin to break down the food you consume into calories, also be aware of the amount of protein, fats, and carbohydrates in everything. The latest recommendations according to the science-based Food and Nutrition Board of the Institute of Medicine's Acceptable Macronutrient Distribution Range (AMDR) are as follows:

Carbohydrates: 45 to 65 percent of your daily calories
Protein: 10 to 35 percent of your daily calories
Total fat intake: 20 to 35 percent of your daily calories[6]

In recent years, I have seen cases of people having trouble losing weight at these numbers. I have concluded a few things. One, they are underestimating how much they are consuming.

Two, they are not metabolizing well due to an untreated hormone condition, a specific medication they take, or a lack of exercise. Remember: the only way to lose weight is to eat less than your body needs. Therefore, if you are accurately consuming very close to the 1500–1800 calorie a day range, depending on whether you are a man or a woman, and you are still not having success losing weight, you'll need to take a very close look in order to fix your problem.

My first suggestion is for you to increase your exercise by 15 minutes a day for a few weeks. If this doesn't help, go visit a doctor and have him or her check out your blood work and hormone levels. In extreme cases, lowering your calorie intake a bit more is the only option. However, this is a last resort and is not generally the solution.

In the next chapter, it's time to dive in to the food. I want to share with you some secrets for getting quality and quantity from your meals!

15

There's a Knock at the Door

I'm not sure if you're like me when it comes to a knock at the door, but if I'm not expecting someone, I sometimes dread answering it. I like to have a heads-up. I like to know who it is on the other side, expecting me to answer. When I open the door, I make a decision.

If it's the UPS man, I just take what he has for me and say goodbye. Our verbal exchange is pleasant and efficient. In other words, he's not coming in for tea and banana bread, but he and I will still have a cordial and quick conversation. Now, if a mother of one of my children's friends is at my door to exchange kids, it's another story. I'll ask her in, chat a few minutes, and then we'll do our business and she'll be on her way. It's not that I don't enjoy her company, it's that our relationship was established for a purpose, to get our kids together. Therefore, it's unlikely we're going to sit down and discuss politics

155

and our pregnancies. However, if one of my close girlfriends, my mom, my mother-in-law, or another family member is at my door, the greeting is altogether different. It's basically a "come on in, make yourself at home" mentality. In other words, "If you're thirsty, you know where to find the glasses. And feel free to sit down and hang out, there's the couch."

I'm sure you're with me so far. When it comes to food, many of our scenarios for handling it are the same. Some foods should be a quick, occasional, and pleasant exchange. Some foods you can feel more comfortable inviting in for frequent visits. And some foods should just be made right at home . . . in your home.

Several years ago, when I used to enjoy regular trips to the bakery, I wouldn't have understood this concept. I would invite some foods in my life just because they looked good to me. Whether or not they could be a potential killer never even crossed my mind. And I thought in order to lose weight I'd need to bolt my mouth shut permanently! So instead, I kept an open door/open fridge policy. Today I have learned, when it comes to food, what to keep outside, what to invite in, and how long it should stay.

I want to take food and break it down for you this way because I believe shifting perspective a bit, like we did with our calorie "math" in the previous chapter, will help to pull some of the emotion out of your food choices. This will also help you do some quick screening when you hear a knock at the door in the future.

Have you ever wondered why everything that's "buy one, get one free" at the grocery store has been processed in a factory? It's because most of it costs less to make than, let's say, raising a cow or growing an orange tree. By describing foods in this manner, I know I run the risk of suggesting you should never buy chips or granola bars. But don't take it this way. I realize every person shops according to their cooking style, budget, and family preferences. However, let the following serve as a guideline for your grocery shopping, meal planning, and personal food choices.

1. Foods that always have a permanent place in your life and you should welcome at all times (family and close friends):
Anything that grows in a tree, sprouts up from soil, or is pre-packaged by nature. Think about what this includes: all fruits, nuts, vegetables, eggs, brown rice, beans, and oats. Now, you should still take into consideration the calories per serving; however, consuming too much of these foods is the least of your worries. I've yet to hear someone tell me they began to gain weight when they started eating apples constantly. These foods should always be hanging around, handy, and the first ones you reach for when you're hungry.

2. Foods that you should invite in for short but regular visits (your child's friend's mother):
What differentiates the foods in this category is their nutritional value. However, you must always take into consideration both moderation and portion control. This is where animal protein comes in, as well as anything that contains at least one of the foods from the above list. This means French fries (potatoes), peanut butter (peanuts), whole-grain breads and cereals (grains), and so on. All dairy products, oils, and dressings fit in here as well. While some foods that fall into this category still go through some sort of process, they are good for you and contain essential fats, fiber, and vitamins. However, read their labels and you will find some are much better for you than others. For example, raisin bran cereal is going to be healthier than yogurt-covered raisins. In addition,

many of your favorites from this list can be prepared in a healthy way and still taste delicious. I will share some meal suggestions with you in a later chapter.

3. Foods that you should be friendly to, but not friends with (the UPS man):

You don't need to slam the door in anyone's face. However, you also don't need to have a long visit with everyone that knocks. The same applies to the foods in this group. Everything that fits here should hang around only for a few seconds—just long enough for you to say hi, have a few bites, and then send it on its merry way. Therefore, anything that goes through a process from start to finish in a factory (think gummy bears), or has an amount of sugar or saturated fat that outweighs any vitamin content or other health benefits should go into this group. Basically: most candies, cookies, baked goods, and ice cream.

Now, as you begin to account for your daily calories, use the guide below to help you with your shopping list. While this list is not complete, it will serve as a regular reference.

Foods That Are Always Welcome

Almonds	Cabbage	Eggs
Apples	Cantaloupe	Grapefruit
Bananas	Carrots	Grapes
Bean sprouts	Celery	Green beans
Berries	Collards	Green or red
Black beans	Corn	peppers
Broccoli	Cucumbers	Green peas
Brown rice	Dried fruits	Kale

Kidney beans

Kiwi

Lettuce

Mushrooms

Navy beans

~~Old-fashioned oatmeal~~

Onions

Oranges

Peaches

Peanuts

Pears

Pecans

Pineapple

Pinto beans

~~Plums~~

Pumpkin

Soy beans

Spaghetti squash

Spinach

Sweet potatoes

Tofu

Tomatoes

Turnips

Walnuts

Watermelon

White potatoes

Yellow squash

Zucchini

Foods That Can Visit Regularly

All oils

Bagels

Biscuits

Breads

Cereal

Cheese

Chicken

Crackers

Fish

Hummus

Lamb

Muffins

Pancakes

Pita chips

Popcorn

Pork

Red meat, the leaner the better

Salad dressings

Tortillas

Turkey

Yogurt

Foods That Should Come and Go Quickly

All kiddy candy: gummy bears, malted milk balls, etc.

All baked goods: chocolate cake, key lime pie, etc.

Ice cream

Anything that automatically makes you crave more than one bite!

Please remember I have one goal when it comes to teaching you about food and its role in weight loss and weight maintenance, and it's this: I desperately want you to stop seeing food as your enemy and instead have a working knowledge of what to eat and when. I can tell you learning how to fit all foods I love into my life has made all the difference for me in ending the diet drama. No longer do I need to feel guilty because I had a piece of pie on a Saturday night while on a date with my husband. But don't hear me wrong. There is a proper time and place for indulgence. This is why it's wise to have healthy options on hand when a craving for something smacks you in the face and it's a Tuesday afternoon.

I have found protein shakes to be a great choice for a tasty treat. They can serve as a source of solid nutrition without having an excess of empty calories like, for example, a chocolate-chip cookie dough Blizzard would have. In the following chapter, I am going to share with you how to "shake it up" with some fun recipes for making healthy and delicious shakes.

16

Shake It Off!

*F*or years, I skipped breakfast and stayed fat. Back then, I'd regularly scratch my head around noon and then, as hunger would begin to kick in, a "free-for-all" ensued. In other words, let the eating begin!

Harvard says a person is seven times more likely to be overweight if they skip breakfast. A database of people who have successfully lost 50 pounds or more and kept it off for five years or longer shows that 78 percent of its participants eat breakfast.[7]

However, through my own past experience and now through what I hear from many folks I've worked with, I know that breakfast is still a great challenge. If you are reading this and you are a regular breakfast eater, great! However, the point of this chapter is to clue you in on the benefits of using protein shakes as a solid choice. Shakes are a great way to get lots of essential things you need in your daily diet—in a hurry, and in a tasty way. Now, I'm not talking about a Frosty from Wendy's. The shakes I'm talking about need to have a solid balance of protein, fats, and carbohydrates.

I used to call these kinds of shakes protein shakes. But the truth is, this implies a very high protein content and doesn't emphasize any other ingredient. So now I'd rather call them "smart shakes."

Basically any shake you whip up that has a ratio close to 40 percent protein, 30 percent carbohydrates, and 30 percent fat is a smart shake. Oh, one more thing: it should be around 350 calories, but no more than 400 if you are trying to maintain your weight, and no more than 300 calories for weight loss. The calorie content in a shake can add up quickly based on the ingredients you use. So watch out! For your information, all of the recipes here are between the 250–300 calorie range.

Also, in the recipes I'm going to share, you will note the need for a scoop of protein powder. This gets you the protein amount you need in the shake in a form you can blend to be drinkable. I've never been one for drinking raw eggs! As far as the brand of protein you choose, be sure it is low in carbohydrates and fat. You'll want to try to add those to your shake with ingredients that are solid—not powdered.

I try to make the shake-making process fun for my whole family. Be creative and try to dream up a signature shake everyone in your house will enjoy! Here are a few of my favorites to get you started.

Each of these recipes makes one shake. Unless the recipe says otherwise, simply toss all ingredients in your blender and blend away!

Nice (Not Naughty) Pumpkin Spice

1 scoop	vanilla protein powder
¼ c.	pumpkin puree
1 c.	skim milk or soy milk
½ tsp	pumpkin pie spice
2 packets	sugar substitute
¼ c.	light whipped topping
1 c.	ice cubes

Sweet Home Strawberry-Banana

1	scoop vanilla protein powder
1 c.	skim milk
1	frozen banana
10	frozen strawberries
½ tsp	vanilla
1 packet	sugar substitute

OJ Dream-Sicle

1	scoop vanilla protein powder
½ c.	orange juice
1 c.	skim milk
dash	of orange zest
1 packet	sugar substitute

Just Like Cherry Pie Minus a la Mode

1 scoop	vanilla protein powder
4–5	maraschino cherries
1	small container Dannon Light and Fit Cherry-Vanilla Yogurt
½ sheet	low-fat graham cracker
1 c.	ice

Peachy-Tea Time!

1 scoop	vanilla protein powder
1 c.	Crystal Lite peach tea
4–6 slices	frozen peach
1 c.	low-fat vanilla yogurt
1 packet	sugar substitute
6	ice cubes

Kinda Like Mom's Apple Pie

1 scoop	vanilla protein powder
1	small apple, peeled, cored, and sliced
2 packets	sugar substitute
½ tsp	cinnamon
¼ tsp	nutmeg
1 c.	light vanilla yogurt
½ c.	light apple juice
½ c.	water
8–10	ice cubes

Proof's in the Butterscotch Pudding

1 scoop	vanilla protein powder
2 Tbsp	sugar-free butterscotch pudding mix
½ tsp	vanilla
dash	of cinnamon
½ c.	water
½ c.	skim milk
1 packet	sugar substitute
8	ice cubes

Get-You-Thin-Mint

1 scoop	chocolate protein powder
1 packet	sugar-free hot chocolate mix

1 tsp   mint flavoring
½ c.   skim milk
½ c.   water
  8   ice cubes

Almond-Joyed

1 scoop   chocolate protein powder
  1 c.   skim milk
2 Tbsp   chocolate syrup
  1 tsp   almond flavoring
    15   whole raw almonds
    10   ice cubes

Blend all ingredients except almonds and ice cubes.
Then add nuts and cubes and blend again.

Don't Ya Want S'more?

1 scoop   chocolate protein powder
      2   1-oz squares of dark chocolate (try for at
         least 70 percent cocoa)
      2   marshmallows, cut into pieces
½ sheet   low-fat graham cracker
2 packets   sugar substitute
    1 c.   skim milk

Chocolate Co-Co Ca-Banana

1 scoop   chocolate protein powder
2 Tbsp   sweetened coconut
  1 c.   skim milk
    ½   frozen banana
    8   ice cubes

It's Gonna Make YOU Snicker

1 scoop	chocolate protein powder
2 tsp	unsalted peanuts
1 Tbsp	peanut butter
1 tsp	sugar-free chocolate syrup
2 packets	sugar substitute
1 c.	skim milk
8	ice cubes

Just Call Me Coffee in the Morning!

1 scoop	chocolate protein powder
½ c.	black coffee
½ c.	skim milk
2 packets	sugar substitute
10	ice cubes

Cookies and Cream

1 scoop	chocolate protein powder
10	fat-free chocolate animal crackers
2 tsp	sugar-free chocolate pudding mix
2 packets	sugar substitute
1 c.	skim milk

PB & J Never Goes Away

1 scoop	vanilla protein powder
1 Tbsp	sugar-free vanilla pudding mix
1 c.	skim milk
1 Tbsp	all-fruit strawberry spread
1 Tbsp	crunchy peanut butter
10	ice cubes

Piña Colada Anytime You Wanna

1 scoop	vanilla protein powder
1	small container Dannon Light and Fit Piña Colada Yogurt
½ c.	frozen pineapple chunks
1 Tbsp	sweetened flaked coconut
½ c.	water
8	ice cubes

Just Another Manic-Mango Smoothie

1 scoop	vanilla protein powder
½ c.	ripe mango
dash	of ginger
1 tsp	lime juice
1 tsp	vanilla extract
½ c.	low-fat vanilla yogurt
1 packet	sugar substitute
½ c.	water
10	ice cubes

17

Going Lighter, Getting Flavor

I think making lighter, healthier food choices without sacrificing flavor is one of the most challenging things people face when aiming to improve their diets. Part of the problem is that fat is what makes things taste really, really good, and sugar comes in a close second. Next time you're in the grocery store, take a close look at all the diabetic or low-carb products. You'll find they are nearly all high in fat. And on the opposite side, things marked low-fat often have a high sugar content. Remember, people won't buy something in a package that doesn't taste decent.

The key to getting flavor out of food and still keeping it on the lighter side is to know where natural or healthy flavors can be added, or at least where a lighter ingredient can be substituted. When cooking at home, try to have a good variety of spices and don't be shy about experimenting with them. Also, try using the low-fat options of things such as mayo, salad dressing, sour cream, and even cheese.

Now, in my house, everyone knows Monday through Thursday there will probably not be any red meat. Not because I think all red meat is evil, but because I like to keep dinner simple and low-fat. This means I opt for chicken and turkey most weekday nights. Does this rule ever get broken? Yep. Just last night, in fact. However, I am consistent enough—meaning I stick to my rules for the most part—that no one in my house would ever expect hamburgers on a Tuesday night.

However, Sunday is a very different story. I have had a great time the past few years teaching all my kids to cook. In fact, at this moment my sons seem to enjoy it more than my daughters do. When the weekend rolls around, I will usually bring up the subject of our Family Sunday Splurge dinner. Not that this meal is never on the healthy side; however, if this happens, it's not on purpose. For example, last week was homemade fried chicken, potatoes, and gravy. So the chicken was still there, but the double-deep frying method Jake and I used to cook it definitely counteracted any semblance of nutritional value. And when potatoes have been smothered in heavy cream, butter, and gravy they are a little too good to be good for you. I'm sure you get the point. Consider setting some rules in your home for having a special no-holds-barred meal that everyone can look forward to. And then focus on keeping the rest of your meals lighter. This will provide a meal for everyone to regularly look forward to, and you'll still feel good about what you're serving the majority of the time.

Speaking of time, there is no way to cut calories if you aren't willing to take the time to plan ahead a little. I know how hectic parenting is—getting kids to school, getting homework done, going to soccer practice, serving in your community or church, and running a business at the same time can be crazy. In fact, I'm exhausted just from typing all this.

However, I've learned everything runs much smoother when I am prepared. Not that I try to cook an elaborate dinner for my gang every day during the week. In fact, it's quite the opposite. However, I do try to have about ten standard meals in my back pocket that are healthy, flavorful, and quick. This serves two purposes. One, I am able to shop for many of the same standard things each week, and two, I don't need to scramble at the last second and settle for a drive-thru dinner.

I'm going to share five of these go-to meals with you. However, please check my website at www.faithfoodandfitness.com for more recipes and ongoing updates.

You will notice one meal looks like breakfast. But who says an omelet can't be eaten at dinner? Try it sometime. It's really easy, really delicious, inexpensive, and quick!

Turkey Meatballs Marinara and Angel Hair Pasta

Serves four

Meatballs

1 lb	ground turkey
1 c.	Italian breadcrumbs
¼ c.	extra virgin olive oil
2	eggs
1 Tbsp	Italian seasoning
2 Tbsp	chopped fresh garlic
pinch	of salt
dash	of pepper

Marinara

1	green pepper
1	red pepper
1	onion

1	32 oz. can crushed tomatoes
1	32 oz. can tomato sauce
2 Tbsp	chopped garlic
3 Tbsp	Italian seasoning
1	bay leaf
1 tsp	salt
1 tsp	pepper
1 lb	whole wheat angel hair pasta

First, preheat oven to 400 degrees. Next, mix all the meatball ingredients together. It's a good idea to use your hands so all the flavors are well mixed. Next, roll the meatball mix into two-inch balls and line them up on a baking sheet. Bake for about 20 minutes. To check doneness, cut through one to make sure the meat is white. Be sure not to overcook them; they can become dry.

Chop peppers and onion, and lightly sauté them in a tablespoon of olive oil. Next, combine your tomatoes and seasonings in a pot and stir in your sautéed vegetables. At this point, you may need to add a cup of water to keep the sauce from becoming too thick.

Cook sauce on a medium heat for about 30 minutes, adding in the fully cooked meatballs for the last 10 minutes.

After you add the meatballs to the sauce, bring a pot of salted water to a boil to cook your pasta. Angel hair pasta is usually done in 6–8 minutes; next, add a handful of ice cubes to stop the cooking and drain pasta. Serve with marinara and meatballs.

Try adding a bright green salad!

Ginger-Honey Glazed Barbecued Chicken with Brown Rice

Serves four

⅓ c.	honey
⅓ c.	low-sodium soy sauce
⅓ c.	rice vinegar
2 cloves	garlic, crushed
1 Tbsp	freshly grated ginger
2–3 lbs	skinless, boneless chicken breasts

Begin by combining the honey, soy sauce, vinegar, garlic, and ginger in a small saucepan. Cook over high heat until the mixture reduces by half. Let cool. Next, spray your grill with non-stick spray (or oil it well) and preheat grill to medium-high. Season the chicken breasts with salt and pepper. Proceed to grill the chicken until it's fully cooked, turning once. Brush breasts on both sides with the honey mixture, then grill 2 to 3 minutes more on each side.

Prepare 2 cups of brown rice, using the directions provided on the bag.

Finally, drizzle the chicken breasts with the remaining honey mixture and serve with a half cup of brown rice.

Veggie Cheesy Omelet

Serves four

4	eggs
1 c.	liquid egg substitute, such as Egg Beaters
½ c.	low-fat milk
6	cherry tomatoes, halved
1	scallion, sliced

  1 c.　baby spinach, washed, with water still
　　　　clinging to leaves
  ¼ c.　onion, chopped
  ½ c.　broccoli, chopped
  2 Tbsp　extra virgin olive oil
  ½ c.　reduced-fat cheddar cheese
  ⅛ tsp　salt
  ⅛ tsp　freshly ground pepper
  1 Tbsp　water

(Note: you can pretty much add any veggies you want to this omelet, just be sure your egg mixture isn't overpowered.)

First, begin by chopping all your veggies. Next, beat your eggs, Egg Beaters, and milk together in a large bowl. Add 1 Tbsp oil to a small nonstick skillet and heat over medium-high heat. Add veggies and sauté for 1 to 2 minutes. Remove half of veggies and set aside. Next, pour half of the egg mixture into the skillet, reduce heat to medium-low, and continue cooking, stirring constantly with a heatproof rubber spatula, until the egg begins to set, about 20 seconds. Continue cooking, lifting the edges so the uncooked egg will flow underneath, until mostly set, about 30 seconds more. Sprinkle half of the cheese, salt, and pepper over the omelet. Lift up an edge of the omelet and drizzle the tablespoon water under it. Cover, reduce heat to low and cook until the egg is completely set and the cheese is melted, about 2 minutes. Fold in half using spatula. Repeat this process for the second omelet, beginning by adding the remaining Tbsp of oil to the skillet. Cut each folded omelet in half, and serve with one whole-grain English muffin and a small bowl of fresh fruit.

Honey Mustard Chicken Strips and Sweet Potatoes

Serves four

¾ c.	light soy sauce
⅔ c.	honey
⅓ c.	dry sherry
½ tsp	garlic powder
¼ tsp	ground ginger
1½ lbs	fresh asparagus spears
6	boneless, skinless chicken breast halves, cut into ¼-inch strips
¼ c.	stone-ground mustard
2 Tbsp	sesame seeds, toasted
3	medium tomatoes, cut into wedges
8 c.	mixed salad greens
	honey mustard dressing
2	baked sweet potatoes

First, stir together first five ingredients; set ½ cup of the mixture aside. Next, pour remaining soy sauce mixture evenly into two heavy-duty zip-top plastic bags. Snap off tough ends of asparagus, and place asparagus spears in one bag. Add chicken strips to remaining bag. Seal and refrigerate at least two hours.

Next, drain chicken and asparagus, discarding marinade. Place chicken on a lightly greased roasting pan. Place asparagus in a lightly greased 9 x 13 pan. Stir together your reserved ½ cup of soy sauce mixture, mustard, and sesame seeds. Pour ½ cup of this mixture over chicken, and the remaining ¼ cup over the asparagus.

Bake chicken at 425 degrees for 5 minutes. Add asparagus to oven, and bake chicken and asparagus for 10 minutes. Arrange chicken, asparagus, and tomato wedges over salad greens, and drizzle with honey mustard dressing. Serve with half of a baked sweet potato.

Roasted Lemon-Pepper Chicken with Nutty Rice

Serves four

1	whole chicken
2 Tbsp	olive oil
1 tsp	thyme
1 tsp	rosemary
1 tsp	lemon-pepper seasoning
1 tsp	salt
2 c.	cooked brown rice
½ c.	toasted pecans
½ c.	dried cranberries

Pre-heat oven to 350 degrees. Line a roasting pan with aluminum foil. Next, mix all seasonings in a small bowl. Prepare chicken by rubbing first with olive oil and then with the dry seasoning mixture.

Place chicken in roasting pan and bake for about 45 minutes or until fully cooked.

Combine cooked rice with the pecans and cranberries. Add salt and pepper to taste, and serve with a vegetable like steamed broccoli or green beans. Enjoy!

Dining Out without Caving In

While fast-food is at the bottom on my list when it comes to quality, for some people there is no escaping it from time to time, so I went through some menus and picked what I feel are some decent choices (note this is with no condiments—don't forget to factor them in).

McDonald's

Grilled Chicken Classic	420 Calories
Southwest Salad with Grilled Chicken	320 Calories
Egg McMuffin	300 Calories
Regular Cheeseburger	300 Calories

Burger King

BK Veggie Burger	420 Calories
Whopper Junior	370 Calories
Ham, Egg, and Cheese Croissan'wich	340 Calories
Eight Piece Chicken Tenders	370 Calories

Subway

6-Inch Oven Roasted Chicken Breast	315 Calories
6-Inch Subway Club	320 Calories
Veggie Delight Wrap	330 Calories

Wendy's

Jr. Bacon Cheeseburger	320 Calories
Chili	280 Calories
Ultimate Grilled Chicken Filet	320 Calories

Taco Bell

Bean Burrito	350 Calories
Crunchy Supreme Taco	200 Calories
Chicken Chalupas	300 Calories

18

Muscle Really Matters

here is no way I can help you walk stronger, look better, and feel fabulous without discussing the value of gaining muscle. I know some folks are so accustomed to watching their weight closely on a scale that the concept of trying to add something doesn't really make much sense to them. If you have been one of these people, it's okay. Don't worry. It's not my goal to help you add weight. Instead, I'm going to talk about how to begin to lose weight by adding muscle. Please read on to discover the irony in this physiological process.

First, learn muscle's job! The primary purpose of muscle is to cushion and protect our bones so we have physical stability and mobility. Now, don't forget, fat is also there to help do this. Also, both fat and muscle store energy. Even the world's leanest body builder or fastest marathoner will still have some body fat.

Which one has the ability to get stronger, muscle or fat? That's right . . . it's your muscles. I've yet to hear someone say they're going to the gym to "work out their fat." Work *off*, maybe. This is because the properties of fat make it mushy and undesirable, while strong muscles have a nice aesthetic appeal.

However, when it comes to losing weight, the importance of strength training and building muscle is an issue of metabolism. The more lean muscle a person has on their body, versus fat, the more quickly they will metabolize calories. This is because muscle needs more calories to function than fat.

Once a person hits his or her mid-twenties, their muscle mass begins to decline by as much as half a pound a year. This is why a teenager can afford to eat more calories than a forty-year-old, even if both have the same level of daily activity. However, if that person in his or her forties has done a good job working to maintain their muscle, they could have the metabolism of a twenty-year-old!

It's funny. Every year millions of women will spend lots of time, energy, and money on new tricks that promise to make them look younger, when in reality it's your age on the inside that matters most when it comes to long life and quality living. Strength training is the cheapest and most effective way to reverse the aging process. And while you may think the age of your insides doesn't show up on your outside, don't be so sure. Have you ever noticed a thin, hunched over elderly woman with a rounded belly? Hormone shifts and aging metabolism take the fat from our faces and other spots and begin transferring it to our midsection.

Lifting weights is also a lot safer than going under the knife, and it's much cheaper. Try to imagine the millions of dollars that would be saved on plastic surgery if more people would try strength training!

But what, exactly, is strength training?

Strength Training: A method of improving muscular strength by gradually increasing the ability to resist force through the use of free weights, machines, or the person's own body weight. Strength training sessions are designed to impose increasingly greater resistance, which in turn stimulates development of muscle strength to meet the added demand.[8]

Most importantly, here's what having this improved muscle equals:

More Muscle = Fewer Injuries

More Muscle = Faster Metabolism

More Muscle = Higher Energy Level

More Muscle = Improved Posture

More Muscle = More Self-Confidence

More Muscle = Stronger Bones

More Muscle = Better Fitting Clothes

More Muscle = Healthier Skin

More Muscle = Efficient Heart Function

More Muscle = Chocolate More Often!

Before I share the simple strength training program I've designed for you to use with the Walk with Him program, we need to get a few more things out of the way: EXCUSES! Every one of these listed below I have either used myself or heard from someone else. Information is powerful. Once we know something, we can't say we didn't do it because we didn't know we had to. Trust me. Once I've handed out the chore list at my house and provided the cleaning supplies, the house needs to get clean or someone gets in trouble! Take a close look at these "reasons" for not strength training, and then read on!

Why I Don't Strength Train

1. I Don't Know How

This is totally understandable. Most people need someone to teach them how to read, ride a bike, and tie their shoelaces too. I remember being afraid to ask for help back when I was learning about strength training. The great news is, because I finally did, I can be here to help you now!

2. I Need to See Immediate Results

Yeah, I do too. But the key is to define your results. If you are looking to see nice definition in your arms and legs in a few weeks, I have some not-so-good news: you can't see muscle definition if there are excess fat layers hiding them. This means you need to begin to look for quick results you can control quickly, and long-term results you can control over time. You can make a goal to strength train two times this week. At the end of the week, if you did it, you will get the immediate result of feeling good for sticking to your goal. Make sense?

3. I Have a Fear of Soreness

This one can be valid, especially because muscle soreness can be aggravating, as it can make the simplest things, such as getting up from the toilet, a major chore. Start off slow, but be consistent. Remember, babies would never be born if all women decided their fear of childbirth wasn't worth the joy of giving birth. There is an incredible thrill in getting stronger!

4. I'm Worried about Getting Too Big

I promise, unless you start taking testosterone shots and eating eggs by the dozen, this won't happen! Whether you are a man or a woman, gaining massive amounts of muscle requires massive amounts of calories. People who are in the process of trying to lose weight are generally cutting calories. Therefore, getting "big" isn't possible. And because muscle takes up to five times *less* space than fat, it's also not realistic to turn any fat on your body directly into muscle.

5. I Just Don't Like It

In discussing this one, I could take a few different approaches. For example, I don't like taking showers or getting the wax out of my ears. But I go ahead and do both because I do like being clean. If you want to experience being well, you'll need to strength train anyway—whether you like it or not. However, there are ways to do it that you may find more bearable. You can try group classes, or exercising with a friend, a spouse, or your kids.

6. I Have No Time

Time is such a funny subject. Do you realize it creates more equality among all people than race, gender, age, or height ever could? Think about it. If you are alive, you have the same amount of time as everyone else who is also living. The truth is, we all make time for the things that matter the most to us. I asked my husband once, on Saturday night, if he thought he was going to have time to watch Sunday football . . . and what do you think he said?

7. I'd Rather Just Walk

I'd rather you just walk, also. But we aren't talking about things we'd rather do. Instead, we are talking about things we need to do. I'd rather go grocery shopping than put groceries away. But I need to do both if I want to have food in my fridge. To obtain fitness, you will need to do resistance training.

8. I Can't Afford the Gym

It seems money is tight for most people these days. Having a big family myself, and owning our own business, I certainly understand the need to be on a budget. To strength train effectively, you don't need a gym membership. While it can be helpful for some, it can be quite intimidating for others. If you aren't able to pay for a gym membership, relax. The exercises I'll show you are as simple as it gets.

9. I Think I Should Lose Weight First

This really goes back to how we build muscle. However, as someone who was once quite overweight, I understand the temptation to back down from strength training. This is mostly because, in the past, you may have found out you can often weigh more when you first start doing it. Why incorporate something that seems self-defeating? However, your body is actually just holding on to more water when you introduce resistance training so your muscles get what they need to repair themselves. This is another reason why getting on a scale too often can sabotage what's best for your body.

10. I'm Concerned People Will Think I'm Too Vain

Then you probably think this book is about you! And it is . . . but it's also about God more than anything. The vanity struggle boils down to a matter of motive. Interestingly, I've worked with orthodox Jewish women who believed showing their knees, elbows, or even their collarbone was inappropriate. In their faith, it was a means of perhaps attracting unwanted attention. But these women still sought me out as their trainer, and worked out quite hard. Exercise for them had nothing to do with getting ready for swimsuit season. They would even wear long tops and skirts while we "did our thing." In their hearts, the desire to take good care of the body God had gifted them with was the real priority. Therefore, the concept of vanity when it came to working out wasn't even a consideration for them.

As long as we regularly check out our main motives, we can avoid this issue. Also, don't be overly concerned with what other people think of you anyway. There will always be a jealous few who make you question your sincerity. Let the Lord lead you when it comes to whether you need to readjust why you are doing what you are doing.

Just a Ball

Now that we have all that out of the way, here's the awesome news!

You can begin to strength train two to three times a week, starting today, and with just a ball. In fact, the name of the strength training workout I've designed, which will work beautifully with your walking program, is called JAB (Just a Ball). These exercises are simple, easy to understand, and best of all, can be done anywhere, anytime, with anyone . . . who has just a ball!

For as long as I've been resistance training, I've wanted to develop a workout with a simple piece of equipment that was not only portable, but could also be done outside of a gym. I came up with lots of ideas over the years, and I've also tried many gizmos. But I've finally found nothing trains your body better than your own body. By means of using our own body weight, along with a weighted ball that can range anywhere from 6 to 12 pounds, I have come up with a workout that hits all of our major muscle groups—and is super simple and super fun! Just begin to think about the saying, "I'm having a ball." This will be you, very soon.

I recommend you use these JAB exercises two to three times a week, along with your Walk with Him program. If you are walking early in the morning, try adding them in later in the day for an extra boost to your metabolism. There are ten exercises described here; however, the combinations are endless. For an instructional video for each of these exercises, and many others, visit my website, www.faithfoodfitness.com.

1. **Reach Row**. Begin by placing your feet about a foot wider than shoulder-width apart, holding the ball before you in both hands. Next, slightly bend your knees. Bend at the waist until your back is flat. Reach in front with the ball, arms straight, then pull the ball to one side, back to the front, then to the other side, as if you are rowing a canoe. Complete three sets of 10, 20, and 30.

2. **Twist Tri**. Begin by placing your feet shoulder-width apart. With the ball in both hands, reach straight up. Next, twist your hips to one side, pivoting slightly with both feet, while bending your elbows until the ball is behind your head. Remember to keep your arms close to your ears. Straighten your arms, and return to center front. Do the exercise on each side for three sets of 20.

3. **Swing Chop**. Begin with your feet shoulder-width apart and the ball in both hands resting on your right thigh. Next, swing the ball up toward your left side, while pulling up your right knee at the same time. Bring the

ball fully overhead, then return to your starting position. Do one set of 20. Switch sides. Do one set of 20 on this side. Repeat on both sides twice more for three complete sets.

4. **Squat Drop**. Begin in a forward facing position with your feet just beyond shoulder-width apart. Grip the ball at your chest with both hands, palms facing in. While making every effort to keep your shoulders back and your elbows close to your body, squat down, lowering the ball by straightening your arms, then curling the ball up as you rise from the squat. Complete three sets of 10, 20, and 30.

5. **Lunge Tap**. With the ball in both hands, begin by stepping out with one leg, and lunging back with the opposite leg. Bring the ball to shoulder height in front of you. Next, bend your knees until your rear knee nearly touches the ground, or as far as is comfortable. Keep your weight centered. Be careful not to let your front knee jut out past the toe. This may be a sign you need to take a bigger step or your weight is leaning too far forward. As you reach the bottom of your lunge, drop the ball down until it taps on your front knee. Return to starting position. Complete one set of 15 on each side. Repeat on both sides twice more for three complete sets.

6. **Press Pull**. Lie down flat on your back, knees bent, with the ball in both hands behind your head. Lift your shoulders slightly off the ground. As you pull your knees to your chest, press the ball up and away, bringing it around to reach your knees. Release back to your starting position. Repeat for three sets of 25.

7. **Half-Moon**. Sit straight up on your knees, holding the ball overhead in both hands. Twist to one side, while

creating a half-moon with the motion of the ball. Return to center. Go to the opposite side. Complete for three total sets of 20.

8. **Knee Over.** Lie down flat on your back, with the ball held above your head in both hands. Bend your knees to a 90-degree angle, lifting your feet off the ground and crossing your ankles. Begin to complete a full sit-up; however, bring the ball up and over the top of your knees as you crunch. Return to starting position. Complete a total of three sets of 25.

9. **Side Burn.** Sit up, with both feet flat on the floor and knees bent. Lean back, gripping the ball in front of you. Let your feet come off the floor. Pull your knees in to one side, and bring the ball to the opposite side, until it's at your waist. Return to your starting position, and repeat on other side. Complete a total of three sets of 20.

10. **One-Arm Kickback.** Get on your hands and knees. Keeping your back flat, roll the ball out a few inches in front of you with one hand. Kick back your opposite leg until it is parallel to the ground, with your foot flexed. Return to starting position. Do a total of three sets of 15 on each side.

Part 4

The Win

19

The Truth about Training

*H*ave you ever been a little weirded out when someone you know begins to make a statement, but as they begin, these words come out: "Just to be honest with you"? How about after, when they add, "Really, I'm telling you the truth"? Truthfully, I'm as guilty as anyone. I've lately found myself saying these very things. In fact, I don't dare count how many times I've already done it in this book. In a perfect world, we should never really need to qualify or justify anything we say as being honest or entirely truthful. Right? Unless, of course, we think there is a chance the other person may not believe us. But why wouldn't they? It's because of a little thing called life!

We all form beliefs as to whether something we are being told is truthful based on the reliability of the person who is saying it, on our personal life experiences, or on how we've witnessed someone else face a similar situation and seen their end result. Thanks to this age of information we live in, with the internet, *Oprah*, and *Dateline*, most people these days are now jaded to the point they have trouble taking anyone's word for anything. Subsequently, we all sometimes feel the need to qualify the integrity of our conversations with blankets of reassurance that we are telling the truth.

I'll never forget dropping off my youngest child, Luke, for his first day of kindergarten, at the ripe age of five. I literally fell onto the steering wheel in tears that morning as I was leaving. Yes. I'll admit, I was sad my littlest one was leaving me home—alone. But the clincher was when I looked up and saw the sign on the gate of the school, "You are now entering a drug-free zone." This wasn't great news to me! I kind of assumed it was a drug-free zone back when I registered him for school. *Gee, now that you've told me it is, I'm now afraid my son is going to need to "Just say no" before his first school day is done! Fabulous.*

Don't worry, I did make a phone call, and there had never been a drug problem at his elementary school. *Hooray?* However, during my chat with the administrator, he told me the sign I was calling about was a simple matter of the school board trying to reassure parents. I shared my concern. I told him the sign raised a red flag for me. He responded that it was better to raise a red flag that indicated a remote possibility than to say nothing and allow any parent to feel nervous saying goodbye to their precious little ones.

After my chat, I realized whether the sign was there or not was irrelevant. God was Luke's ultimate protector. Sure, the sign challenged my belief he was safe and intimated he might be in jeopardy. However, the reality is the warning didn't protect or expose him in any way. The proclamation was just that, a bold statement offering reassurance. And for some people, especially someone who was perhaps exposed to drugs at an early age, the sign may deliver a sense of security. Let's face it. No one wants to hear a statement that indicates potential harm. We'd rather just walk around feeling warm and fuzzy when it comes to most things in life. I mean, have you every really studied the potential side effects when you reach for a Tylenol? It seems so much nicer just to take one to get rid of a headache than to read the bottle and worry about getting liver disease.

However, our safety and security would never exist if we had no knowledge of risk. When an outcome is critical, assurance is insurance. When I went to board a plane a few weeks after 9/11, I was happy to comply with all the extra security measures. However, if the airport had decided to implement the same rules a month before the attack, we would all have been complaining like crazy.

Training your body, soul, and spirit to walk with God requires sacrifice. It will challenge you in every way. I don't say this as a red flag; instead, I want you to have assurance in the outcome. This way, down the road, when this book begins to collect dust (hopefully it won't, as it sits just under your Bible) you'll remember the information in this chapter and it will help you breathe a sigh of relief.

The Sacrifices of Training to Walk with Him

I have learned there is a smart way to train, and then there's my way. My way is smart only when I allow God to be my trainer. By nature, I wake up and want to accomplish everything on my list by 9:00.

191

Some days I rise, and hear the Lord whisper, *Good morning, daughter*. And I respond, *Good morning, Savior*. Other days, I wake up and I hear, *You're welcome*.

However, it's somehow now dinnertime and we've just said a blessing over our meal.

If you and I don't choose to begin each day by asking God to walk with us, we run the risk of regular injury. It's not necessarily the kind that will prohibit us from exercise, meaning it won't always be physical injury. My definition of an injury is anything that threatens my ability to complete any task at any level less than my very best. Trying to do life each day without the Lord makes us vulnerable to sitting on the sidelines of life.

Know the Sacrifices, Savor the Victories

Sacrifice and victory go hand in hand. In fact, no victory could ever feel like "victory" without some measure of sacrifice. As you begin to walk more, there are guaranteed to be days when you just don't feel like it. In the world of business, an acronym used often is ROI. It stands for "return on investment." You see, anyone who is seeking to own a successful company would put money only into a concept if they had the complete conviction it would deliver not only their initial investment, but much more. The Walk with Him program has the potential to be the greatest investment of your lifetime.

There isn't a better way to look at sacrificial living than to see it through the life of Jesus. Although we can never live a sin-free life, Jesus offers us the example of His life in order to show us the realm of possibilities—if we will exercise our faith in Him to sustain us. The sacrifices of Jesus can directly apply to any success we seek in life. If you want to walk stronger, be healthy, and be more effective for His kingdom, think about "what did Jesus do?" And as you continue on your Walk with Him journey, rest assured there is nothing you'll feel or face that He hasn't already conquered!

Jesus Sacrificed Comfort

Going all the way back to His birth, Jesus sacrificed comfort (see Luke 2). A manger isn't exactly a high-end, hand-carved, imported Italian crib. Imagine—the Savior of the world, who could have rightfully requested a grand entrance complete with pomp and circumstance—chose a manger. As a mom, I can't imagine laying my newborn down in a feeding trough for livestock. (But then, I can't fathom giving birth in a stable, either, with only my husband as my medical team.)

Let's face it, we all want to be comfortable. Recently, I went to speak to a group of missionaries preparing to head out into foreign fields. The training center I arrived at was lovely, but somewhat primitive. I was escorted to my room and immediately I felt like I was camping. There was no television. No internet. Just a single bed with a thin blanket and a small pillow. I was a tad bit aggravated. I immediately began to think about my compromised sleep and that I'd be missing *American Idol*.

Within a few minutes I felt God knocking on my heart: *Remember why you're here*. Then I thought about the real purpose behind my trip. I came to share hope and the faithfulness of God in every situation.

I'm learning all the time how a willingness to sacrifice comfort is one of the greatest testimonies of authentic faith I can display. Can you imagine if I had gotten to the missionary training center and balked—then asked to be taken to a nice hotel? The people who set this up would have questioned if they had chosen the right woman to speak. Also, the missionaries would have heard a message filtered through a selfish heart. If walking with God is something you really want to do, be willing to be uncomfortable from time to time. You'll find supernatural strength in the process.

Jesus Wasn't Afraid to Get Dirty

The picture is a powerful one. Imagine it's the last supper before Jesus is going to die. I have no doubt Jesus didn't bother requesting a last meal of fish tacos or something equivalent. All of the disciples are there, and their feet are covered in dust and dirt from taking the journey to the upper room. And during the meal, Jesus does something remarkable. He gets up and begins to pour water into a basin. Not to rid Himself of germs, but to rid the disciples of their future pride. He proceeds to wash their feet one by one, knowing full well He is going to die soon and that one of these men is going to deny Him and another has already betrayed Him. Jesus wasn't above getting dirty (see John 13:1–17).

The whole image has the power to take your breath away. Jesus teaches us the ultimate display of humility. Do you think He questioned any of them, "Seriously, guys, why are your feet so filthy?" Doubtful. In fact, Jesus likely found the most joy in cleaning the dirtiest. The real question in the end was left up to the disciples: Would they be willing to follow in His footsteps?

To live better, we must be willing to do things from time to time that require us to get dirty. When I initially began attempting to gain control over my weight, I regularly became frustrated. I didn't like "having" to sweat, or "having" to give up certain foods. It just didn't seem fair. I can remember thinking, *Why me? Why is being fat my deal?* But as I imagine the scene at the Last Supper, when Jesus did something He didn't "need" to do, I get it. If He was willing to roll up His sleeves to show His sincerity, why can't I? If you are fully engaged and committed to taking care of your body, getting dirty will be one of the first steps.

Jesus Gave Up His Time

We know our Creator wants us to take a break. In Genesis, He calls for a day of rest. Remember, the fourth commandment is about keeping the Sabbath day holy. So interestingly, why did Jesus let us know He healed people on the Sabbath? There are several places in the New Testament when this takes place.

When challenged, He answered this very question. After the Pharisees voiced their concern, Jesus responded, "Which is lawful for a man to do on the Sabbath, to do good or to do evil, to save life or to kill?" (see Mark 3:1–6). Know this: any time we set out to make a difference with our life, there will be regular time conflicts. Things are going to come up regularly, and physical exhaustion will whisper in our ears.

What it comes down to is our priorities. There are going to be times when we must give up our "free time" in order to save our lives. Gaining and maintaining physical wellness requires this on a regular basis. This is not to say rest isn't vital. However, use wisdom when it comes to what you think you should be doing, and what you really need to do. If you don't take the time to make your wellness a priority, you won't have the strength to encourage others to seek their own healing.

Jesus Didn't Try to Do It Alone

As Jesus began His ministry time on earth, He knew the importance of getting help (see Matt. 4). This is why He assembled the apostles. It's interesting to read the fishing story in Matthew. Jesus was deliberate and uninhibited. Here, Andrew, James, and John are having trouble catching fish. To their surprise, Jesus begins to give them some expert advice. Now remember, He was a carpenter and *they were anglers*. The irony of the story is what happens after they take His advice. They begin to pull in fish everywhere!

There is a time for all of us to let go of inhibition and ask for help. Along your journey, a day is going to arrive when you will need outside support. Remember, the disciples were entering uncharted territory. They had to be a bit nervous about taking such a giant leap of faith and making a major career change.

Jesus taught us that change is a necessary part of life. And to do this, we all will need to sacrifice our inhibitions regularly. Ask yourself: *Will I risk everything I have at this moment to gain everything I could ever need for eternity?* Then ask yourself this: *Will I ask for support along the way?*

Jesus Didn't Feel Like It

He went on a little farther and bowed with his face to the ground, praying, "My Father! If it is possible, let this cup of suffering be taken away from me. Yet I want your will to be done, not mine." (Matt. 26:39 NLT)

Do you realize what this verse means? It means Jesus was anxious. Anxiety is not a sin. What would be sinful is to refuse to do God's will because of it.

I have anxiety often. Probably a little too often (just trying to keep it real). I'll never forget the night before I had my daughter Kayla. Due to previous complications with my first child, I was scheduled to have a C-section. Did you know that knowing what you are about to experience can be much more difficult than simply being thrown into it? It's because of time. You are able to anticipate the outcome. I stayed awake the entire night before I had Kayla, just lying there with my eyes wide open, praying I would go to sleep and wake up with a new baby in my arms. But it didn't go down that way. In fact, the doctor was a few hours late showing up for surgery. It's perfectly normal to feel uneasy about something you know you need to do. But when this happens, follow the lead of Christ. Pray. Have a little talk with God. Speak out your fear. Plead with Him for peace and strength. It will not only make it bearable, but you will begin to feel His hand tightly holding on to yours.

20

Stop. Look. And Listen.

I want to talk to you a bit about the deeper effect walking can have on your life. If you will learn to stop, look, and listen often, walking has the power to deliver a more keen awareness of the world around you.

I love the way Paul Johnson, a historian, talks about the manner in which Jesus walked. In his book *Jesus*, Johnson reminds us that what Jesus looked like is not nearly as important as understanding what He looked at.

> In short, there is no reliable evidence of what Jesus looked like. On the other hand, we know certain things about His visual personality, which struck eyewitnesses and so are recorded in the Gospels. Jesus was very observant. It is notable how many times he is described as looking, looking upon, looking round, looking up. His habit of penetrating observation punctuates the narrative: He was a man greatly interested in detail. He missed nothing. He had a penetrating gaze, which eyewitnesses

noticed and remembered. His all-seeing eyes were, almost certainly, the first thing that struck people about Him.[9]

Have you ever wondered what is the first thing that strikes someone about you? I've met many people whose physicality seemed irrelevant next to their energetic spirit. And I will spend lots of time with them before I even notice they have blue eyes. Then there are some folks who portray an obsession with their appearance, and therefore it's natural to focus on their features.

I go walking at a park near my house several times a week. This park also happens to be the location for my regular "Faith, Food, and Fitness" community outreach workouts. So, basically, it's my home away from home. The only problem with this dream location is the hundreds of ducks that are taking over. It's gotten to the point where traffic coming in can be at a standstill for several minutes while the car at the front of the line is trying to gently usher a pack of ducks safely across the street. (Not to mention they go to the bathroom all over the grassy areas where we work out.) The duck drama would likely be minimal if people would simply stop feeding them. When someone shows up with a bag of bread, these birds flock as if they haven't eaten in weeks. I've even witnessed some pretty major scuffles between them, including biting, and all for a few handfuls of mozzarella cheese one lady brought as part of her own "be kind to animals" campaign.

One week, I had finally had it. It's not that I am a natural killjoy. Far from it! Instead, I was ready to be a solid citizen in my community. In my opinion, when you see a sign that says, "Do Not Feed the Ducks," there is likely a valid reason for adhering to it. And if someone happened to not understand what the sign meant, or they missed seeing it, I decided it would be my self-appointed obligation to educate them accordingly.

I was on my third lap walking around the soccer field when the first opportunity arose to carry this out. I came upon a woman with dark hair I had seen breaking the "duck feeding law" at least a dozen times. I decided at first I'd take a laid-back approach. As I began to a walk alongside her, I simply smiled. Trust me. While it may have appeared genuine, in my mind, it was more a matter of getting her to acknowledge me before I informed her our neighborhood park was not a petting zoo! She nodded back, said good morning, and I then took the cue and struck up a conversation. After a few exchanges about the weather, family, and church, I decided the duck situation needed addressing. After all, I might have trouble telling her to stop feeding them if she and I became too friendly.

I think my transition line went something like this: "So, I've noticed you have quite a thing for the ducks." To this she responded, "Yes, they are my babies!" Now, I don't know about anyone else, but ducks hardly seem like a substitution for a child. I mean, they aren't cuddly, and they don't even cry or giggle. But I wanted to give her the benefit of the doubt. So I said, "Wow. At least there are no diapers to change." She laughed. Then she tried to clear things up for me. "No, you don't understand; my babies helped to save my life." Just before I called the funny farm to come and pick her up, I asked her what she meant.

She then told me the previous year had been the toughest she had ever experienced. She had been diagnosed with stage-four breast cancer and had undergone extensive treatment. Coming to the park each day to see her ducks gave her something to look forward to. She even said that taking care of them had delivered the hope she needed. Hmm. It goes without saying, however, that I felt about an inch small. Give or take a centimeter. After she had poured out her heart, I didn't have the nerve to discuss the posted signs that, if she had adhered to, might have caused her to slip into a deadly depression. Instead, my new friend and I went on to walk a few miles and talk about how good God is!

If we will stop, look, and listen on more occasions during some of our walks, the potential to encourage someone and deepen our human connections will soar. Plus, we may be an answer to someone else's prayer that day.

Why to Stop, What to Look for, and How to Listen

Why to Stop

When I first started driving at age sixteen, I'll never forget some smarty-pants telling me, as I left the agency with my license in hand, not to forget that "Stop signs with a white border around them are optional!" What did I know? I thought this was a friendly tip. The next week, when I noticed the first one with a border, I decided to go ahead and exercise my option. As I approached the four-way stop, I eased through it gently, and decided to make the other cars wait for me. In my mind, "the all-powerful road sign committee" regularly assigned one corner to have a special stop sign. Miraculously, I survived.

However, the honking and hand signals from all the other cars did make me take a closer look at the next hundred or so stop signs. Shockingly, they all had white borders! Just imagine if I had never heard the suggestion to pay close attention to the white borders. I would never have imagined this so-called optional stop sign even existed.

Of course, it didn't take me long to realize I'd been had. But I did learn something—in addition to the fact that all stop signs have white borders. I learned the benefits of paying attention.

In life, we need to stop regularly as if our very lives depend on it. Often they do—and not just while we're driving. My walk with the duck woman made me keenly aware of this. Imagine if I had just stopped and barked at her, "Please stop feeding them!" Whether she would have decided my suggestion was worth listening to would have been irrelevant. I would have been the one who missed hearing her story. So many times, we think stopping is going to cost us something. We start out on a walk with the intention of just getting it over with. However, in reality the calories we are burning and the heart conditioning we are getting are more or less just add-ons to the bigger picture of what could be taking place.

When to stop is something only you can answer. There have been a few times I may have wasted the opportunity to burn off a few more calories by chitchatting for too long with a fellow "walker." But more often than not, I've learned when to stop, and also when to move on. These days I stop when I feel like it the least, and when I want to be alone the most. It seems I can hear God whisper loud and clear by listening to the people He puts in my path at these times.

For those who walk in an area where there isn't much traffic, don't think this message isn't for you. I imagine there are likely many other places you frequent where *to stop* or *not to stop* is an option. Whether you're walking into the post office or around the grocery store, you can still begin to be more aware of opportunities to stop.

What to Look For

After you stop, what you are looking for can be the next challenge. A few years ago, I spent some time studying the presence of angels among us. I went around for about a month looking to meet them in my ordinary life. After all, Hebrews

12:2 tells us to be aware, because we will entertain angels without even knowing it. I figured this meant I could know it, if I were more aware—but after what happened, I realized the whole point is to not know it!

I met a nice woman while I was getting my son a bagel at the local deli one day. She struck up a conversation, saying I looked familiar. Apparently, she had spotted me at church a few weeks prior. I walked away after this exchange thinking, *What a lovely, Christian, grandmother-type.* A few days later, I saw her pumping gas next to me. A few days after that, I was at Starbucks in the mall with a girlfriend, and take a guess at who showed up and sat down beside me. Yes. By this point, after running into her three times in one week (think Trinity/three parts/not a coincidence), I was ready to let her know I was on to her.

I decided to bring up the subject of marriage. An angel couldn't possibly be married, right? However, she was wearing a ring on her left hand, and on the correct finger. I asked her how long she had been married. She responded (you need to believe me), "I've been married to Jesus for as long as I can remember." Was there anything else she needed to say at this point? Apparently there was. About ten seconds later, she said, "I'm also married to Buddha and Muhammad."

Say what? I was so mad. There should be a law against tricking people into thinking you are an angel when in reality you are insane. I immediately said goodbye—and decided my looking skills needed some improving.

When you stop in life, and decide to look around, don't look for a hidden message. Why would God need to hide? If I am entertaining an angel, the whole point is for me not to know it's happening!

Instead, stop along the way and look for the beauty in hearing someone else's miracle story, or look for the pain in their eyes that says "Please pray for me." What we all need to look for is often a matter of not looking too hard. We will overlook the obvious if we try to read between lines that don't exist, and we can miss hearing what God wants to say through the simplest of exchanges.

How to Listen

Learning how to listen is critical. Let's picture you, out walking. You decide to stop, and you look for the obvious reason you're having this encounter. Finally, you'll need to listen. Listening is very hard for me. I love to hear myself talk. And I'm pretty sure others do as well. After all, they never ask me to quit. Then again, they have only about 2.2 seconds to do it while I take an occasional breath.

Yet when I think about it some of my most interesting conversations, and those which have also ministered to me the most, end up involving much more listening on my end. Maybe it's because all the talking I often feel the need to do has already taken place in my head. At some point it can start to sound a little repetitive.

Listening to someone while you walk will require regular eye contact and genuine responses. If I'm involved in a conversation and it's beginning to feel like a waste (for example, we're twenty minutes into whether Brad Pitt and Angelina Jolie should have more kids), I'll find a way to change the subject. The longer I live, the less time I am willing to squander on meaningless conversation. In fact, let this always be a main question in the back of your mind: *What is meaningful about the conversation I am having?*

Not that there isn't an appropriate time to talk about the delicious taste of the dark chocolate in my favorite Black-Jack cherry frozen yogurt.

21

Gaining Speed

*O*n your mark, get set, *go!* We've all heard these words at some point. For me, the most memorable time was back when I was about ten. I was a nonathletic chubby girl with a competitive spirit. After scoping out the sport of softball and breaking my ankle while hopping off a bleacher at my first game, I decided to look for a new sport. Swimming seemed like the natural choice.

I began to practice each afternoon. My plan was to get good at holding my breath first. Then I'd work on technique. For my training, I'd go underneath the water and kick off from one side of the pool with the goal of making it to the other side, all in one breath. Eventually, I became pretty good at it. Then the time came for me to test my speed. I challenged my little sister to race me. I knew there was no way she could beat me. After all, this was *my sport*.

I gathered the whole family. Even my Grandma Parrish was visiting. Everyone was on the patio, gathered around the pool, ready to witness history in the making. My mom was in charge of calling the race. I knew she would be fair. I remember hearing the words, "On your mark, get set, go!" and we both kicked off. Next, all I remember was BAM.

You see, for some reason I decided to close my eyes as I took off (likely because I was praying) and as I approached the other side (for some reason I also had my mouth open), my mouth slammed into the concrete and I knocked out a good part of my two front teeth! Between visits to the dentist to fix my smile, and the time I had spent in a cast as a result of watching a softball game, I felt robbed of the confidence to compete in any arena of sports ever again.

A few years into my fitness journey, I decided to get my "feet wet" in sports again. Just not in the pool. I decided to try running. This seemed like a natural choice for a chick who once weighed over 350 pounds. Who would dare disagree? My frame screamed "natural runner." I signed up for a marathon and began training. It didn't take long for me to become quite frustrated with my efforts to become faster. Even though I had lost the weight, my body reminded me I had once carried what equated to "my husband" on my back. Lots of things hurt . . . regularly. As time went on, I had to reassess why speed was relevant.

Here's what you need to know: gaining speed isn't about becoming the fastest. Instead, it's about being regularly challenged to become better. In this chapter, I'm talking about the literal need for you to work on gaining speed. Earlier in the book I laid out a four-week walking program that had built-in speed drills. However, in terms of your ongoing walking program, aim for two of your five weekly workouts to include some sort of speed challenge. No, you're likely not aiming to win a tangible prize. However, you should be seeking regular results.

I want to share my top reasons why gaining speed is important. I will also show you how to apply these practically to your Walk with Him program.

Gaining Speed

Gaining speed:

> Delivers more confidence
> Keeps things exciting
> Helps relieve stress
> Conditions your heart muscle
> Improves your physique

Delivers More Confidence

Do you realize confidence is the key to every challenge you or I will ever take on in life? When you set out to walk faster and you begin to see improvement, the desire to take it a step further kicks in. Getting into this zone is what sets successful people apart from the rest.

First, calculate a one-mile loop in your neighborhood, or plan to use a treadmill to complete this challenge. Pick a day, and walk as fast as you can for an entire mile. Be sure to time it, and find a place to record your time when you are done. Make it your goal to do this mile twice a week for a month, shaving a few seconds off your time, every time.

Keeps Things Exciting

It saddens me when I meet a person in great shape who says exercise is boring. In other words, they do it but they just don't like it. There is no reason you can't get excited about walking. Not only can you take a different route whenever you want, but you can also get jazzed along the way by increasing your speed.

The best way to keep things exciting is to create mini-challenges. For example, if you are out for a 45-minute walk, every 5 minutes pick a spot in the distance and run to it. This will keep your adrenaline in high gear and give you many measurements for a successful speed walk.

Helps Relieve Stress

I can't speak for anyone else; however, my personal stress level can be dramatically reduced from the time I begin a walk to the time it's over. There are many physiological reasons for this, a majority of which are attributed to the enjoyment of "getting it over." Few people will say, when a workout is over, "I wish I could rewind to the beginning." I've seen this at the front desk of a gym when two friends collide, one entering and the other leaving. The one dripping in sweat has a big grin, while the other person just shakes her head with a disposition that reminds me of the old Dunkin' Donuts commercial where the baker rolls out of bed half-asleep, mumbling, "It's time to make the donuts."

Stress reduction is an awesome by-product of exercise. However, increasing your speed while you're doing it will enhance this natural response. With most things in life, more isn't always more, including walking. But try going for a walk for the sole purpose of de-stressing. Make sure you do this on a day when you are feeling especially overwhelmed. As you work to walk faster, periodically take a break and do some deep breathing. Inhale as deeply as you can through your nose, and slowly release the air through your mouth. Then speed up your walk again. I have no doubt you will finish your workout feeling much less stressed than when you started.

Conditions Your Heart Muscle

The higher volume of blood you pump to the heart muscle, the stronger it will become. But why? Well, think about that tight pair of jeans you practically need to lie down to squeeze into. Even though you feel like you can't breathe when you first put them on, eventually, they become bearable. The material in the jeans begins to give to accommodate your body. Your heart works exactly the same way.

When you first begin to increase your speed, you get out of breath. This is the point most people get nervous and slow down drastically. This would be like ripping off the jeans just when you've got them buttoned. While wearing really tight jeans isn't always enjoyable, there is no way to stretch them to fit better unless you wear them for a bit. Conditioning your heart muscle happens when you increase your speed. You'll need to force yourself to tolerate the intensity for short bursts. Begin with 15-second challenges, then move up to 30 seconds, and eventually complete 1- and 2-minute speed drills.

Note: as I mentioned in an earlier chapter, you may want to consider making an investment in a heart-rate monitor. This handy and inexpensive gadget takes the guessing out of how hard you are working and allows you to concentrate on working to get better. While there are many on the market that have lots of bells and whistles, I have found keeping it simple is a smart way to go. In other words, all you really need is for the monitor to provide a number, not make coffee.

Improves Your Physique

To change the shape of your body, you'll need to work to lose fat and gain muscle. I already discussed this in detail, back in the chapter on strength training. You can also improve your muscle definition with speed. The harder you work out, the more calories you will burn. Period. Of course, there is the age-old argument as to where the calories you burn are "coming off" from. I've done a lot of research, and I've reached this conclusion: it doesn't matter! The more overall calories you burn means the more calories you burn—from all sources. In other words, burn as many calories as you can.

As you work harder and use more energy, your body will begin to change for the better. Stubborn fat deposits will begin to melt away as they are called upon more frequently as a fuel source to get your body through an especially tough workout.

The best way to see your physique change is by taking regular measurements. Simply use a tailor's tape measure and record your chest, waist, hip, thigh, and arm circumference. After you have been doing speed workouts for a month solid, recheck them!

I'm quite sure you are ready to get a move on, now. However, there's one more thing. It has to do with your heart. I know I already explained the benefit of speed for conditioning your heart, but I want you to know what this form of training really delivers in terms of the quality of years you are adding to your life. After all, living longer is a solid goal. However, a better goal is to live longer and feel amazing at the same time. Your resting heart rate is an indicator of how efficiently your heart delivers blood and oxygen to your muscles when they aren't under stress. You see, most of us know how quickly we can get out of breath when we start exercising again after taking a break. Therefore, how high your heart rate can get during exercise isn't a true indicator of your overall cardiovascular fitness. However, your resting heart rate is. Typically, the lower your resting heart rate, the more efficient your heart is, whether you are relaxing or exercising.

Everything eventually succumbs to wear and tear. I learned this just recently as I went to replace a worn-out tire. Apparently, they aren't under the same warranty after I've driven thirty thousand miles on them. Now, think about your heart. Let's say it has a finite number of beats assigned to it before it will wear out. You should aim to condition your heart to need fewer beats while at rest, which is most of your life. After all, even an avid exerciser exercises for a short time in relation to the number of hours in their entire lifespan.

Think about it like this: if my resting heart rate is 60 beats per minute and my girlfriend's is 80, her heart is essentially getting more wear and tear than mine every minute that passes—by 20 beats! This means the lower your resting heart rate is (for those with a healthy heart), the more beats you are banking for the future. Speed training for your heart is like regular oil changes for your car's engine. It's essential to insure a long, healthy life.

22

Every Season . . .

I have thoroughly enjoyed having the opportunity to share some of my insights into the world of walking with you. However, I pray my transparency will touch you above all else. Sure, reading about my pounds lost and my newfound fitness should be encouraging. But in deciding what to take away from this book, please allow this message to penetrate even deeper.

Surprisingly, I understand the shift of seasons, even though I have always lived in South Florida where there are few climate changes between hot and hotter. Think Christmas, 80 degrees. A change of seasons happens for me in terms of what's going on in my life—with my kids, my parents, my deadlines, and of course, the National Football League. After all, this season seems to control Keith and the boys most Sunday afternoons for a few months.

I want us to get up close and personal and talk about what matters the most for a few minutes. Back in the '60s a rock band named the Byrds sang a song called "Turn, Turn, Turn." I've often wondered if the world truly understood the origin of their lyrics. They were actually written by King Solomon, the son of David (think Goliath-slayer). Solomon, the wisest man ever to walk the earth, wrote the following:

> To everything there is a season,
> A time for every purpose under heaven:
> A time to be born,
> And a time to die;
> A time to plant,
> And a time to pluck what is planted;
> A time to kill,
> And a time to heal;
> A time to break down,
> And a time to build up;
> A time to weep,
> And a time to laugh;
> A time to mourn,
> And a time to dance;
> A time to cast away stones,
> And a time to gather stones;
> A time to embrace,
> And a time to refrain from embracing;
> A time to gain,
> And a time to lose;
> A time to keep,
> And a time to throw away;
> A time to tear,
> And a time to sew;
> A time to keep silence,
> And a time to speak;
> A time to love,
> And a time to hate;
> A time of war,
> And a time of peace.

What profit has the worker from that in which he labors? I have seen the God-given task with which the sons of men are to be occupied. He has made everything beautiful in its time. Also He has put eternity in their hearts, except that no one can find out the work that God does from beginning to end.

I know that nothing is better for them than to rejoice, and to do good in their lives, and also that every man should eat and drink and enjoy the good of all his labor—it is the gift of God.

> I know that whatever God does,
> It shall be forever.
> Nothing can be added to it,
> And nothing taken from it.
> God does *it*, that men should fear before Him.
> That which is has already been,
> And what is to be has already been;
> And God requires an account of what is past. (Eccles. 3:1–15 NKJV)

We can't walk and win if we don't understand what's truly at stake. And if we don't walk with Him, our lives will become meaningless. I do not say this to offend you, if you're still trying to do life on your own. However, know this: at some point, you will start to wonder *what for?*

I love that, through King Solomon, God gives wisdom. In fact, it was something Solomon specifically requested from the Lord in prayer. The reason God gave wisdom to him was because it was a selfless request. Solomon wasn't asking for a solid-gold chariot. He simply wanted to understand the purpose of life on the deepest levels.

The verse that always seems to stick out the most for me is where Solomon asks, "What profit has the worker from that in which he labors?" (v. 9). Basically, what he's saying is this: Why on earth do we work so hard? And then he goes on to discuss eternal rewards.

If you finish this book and all you've learned is how to utilize walking as a primary means of maintaining a healthy body, then I have squandered your time and trust. I always enjoy talking about heart-rate monitors and the beauty of the morning dew that I see as I head out for a walk on a cool and crisp fall day. But if you don't get to the *why* behind what you do, you'll eventually see it all as meaningless.

Above all else, you can always find meaning in your walking program if you'll utilize the time it gives you to pursue peace. Recently, after a long day of writing, I began to think about an old friend. She and I had been very close for many years, and then one day we weren't. Looking back, I realized I had made a lot of mistakes. I became too busy—perhaps I was overly zealous about my projects—and I imagine there were many more things I did wrong. Either way, I'm sure you get the picture. There were some serious feelings of hurt on both our parts.

Whenever we are living with some sort of unresolved conflict, bitterness easily takes root. Even if there is still love, care, and concern for the other person, on a human level the feeling of being misunderstood is always a hard pill to swallow.

I can honestly say I was way past feeling bitter. And it bothered me. Not because I couldn't see my faults, but because I became overly concerned as to whether she was aware of hers. Finally, I worked up the courage to call her. I wanted to ask one thing: Would she consider meeting me sometime soon to go out for a walk? She said yes. I was thrilled, and not just because I wanted to have my old friend back or because I hoped to have a deep discussion about lessons we'd both learned from our past offenses. I just wanted peace.

Psalm 34:14, Hebrews 12:14, and Philippians 4:2–3 all essentially say the same thing: do whatever is necessary to be at peace with everyone. I don't believe God wants us to do this in an undignified, groveling sort of way, where we apologize for things that never happened. However, I am convinced peace is possible if both parties have just one commonality: goodwill, which is the deep desire to do the right thing.

I want to challenge you to use walking as a means to pursue peace often. You can do this many ways. When you are in the middle of a heated discussion with your spouse, decide to head out the door together to continue the discussion. I'm not saying to drop the disagreement and walk arm in arm with gritted teeth. I do live in the real world. However, something happens when we take ourselves out of our home or "safe place." The freedom to say things that perhaps we shouldn't goes away. I've seen a major disagreement between Keith and I shrink down to a mutual desire for a quick resolution during a 10-minute walk around our neighborhood. And I'm convinced the same fight could have lasted for hours had we stuck it out in our house.

"Go get some fresh air!" This statement also implies the power of taking a walk. When you start to feel overwhelmed by your responsibilities or your kids, get away. Hit the street. We all know the air isn't literally "fresher" out there, but a change in your environment will offer you a fresh perspective.

I also want to challenge you to occasionally go for a walk with your kids, instead of walking to get away from your kids. I have learned many interesting things during a walk about what's going on with my teenage girls. And for the record, walking in a shopping mall doesn't count.

Here's how walking promotes peace:

1. It's an Instant Ice-Breaker
   * Basically, there is no downtime to feel awkward, like there is if you're sitting across from someone waiting for food. As soon as you start walking, the pace and scenery create instant conversation.
2. It's Private
   * I don't know about you, but I don't always want to be around lots of people when I need to resolve something with one individual. When you go for a walk, you can pick a place that has limited noise.
3. It's Cheap
   * There is no worry as to who's going to pick up the tab. A walk is a totally free way to congregate with another person.
4. It's Rewarding
   * There aren't many ways to spend time with someone that deliver dual rewards. When you walk with someone, not only are you promoting a peace-filled relationship, you are also reaping the reward of exercise. You'll both feel more positive and energized.
5. You're Trapped . . . In a Good Way
   * When you're walking to resolve conflict or to pursue peace, you're trapped with nowhere else to go! The truth is, once you set out, heading in a certain direction, at some point you'll need to turn around. When you are on the phone, you can choose to hang up. When you are in a house, you can choose to leave. But when you're on a walk, you've got to get back. This can be a forced means of communication.

I did end up meeting my old friend down by the beach for a walk. It felt strange at first. I forgot to bring change for the parking meter. She immediately found a bunch of quarters in her car and stuck them in for me. We hugged. That felt strange too. So much had changed since we'd last seen each other. Immediately I asked about her kids. She chuckled as she began to talk about her son. It seemed like only a few years ago I had planned a baby shower for her. Now that child was fifteen years old, stood at 6'5", and was a high school track-and-field star.

As the walk progressed, seven miles later we finally made it back to our vehicles. Just before we said goodbye, she reminded me that she loved me and wished me well. I said the same. And that was it.

Seriously. There was no tearful, "But when you said . . . it made me feel . . ." And that was good. We need to get to the point where we can seek peace without needing to make a point. Thankfully, my friend was on the same page as me, which is why it worked so beautifully. However, there are going to be times when someone in your life will have no desire to reciprocate your goodwill. That's okay. The best part of goodwill comes when you give it without conditions. It becomes a seed planted in the other person's mind, and the more goodwill you show them, the more you will be watering that seed.

You'll have more internal peace and peaceful relationships if you will let seasons come and go instead of constantly trying to fight their beginning or ending. Try to simply anticipate the next arrival. I'd never have the space for some of the awesome friendships I have at this moment if I had fought God and not allowed Him the space to bring a new season of special folks into my life.

23

Staying the Course

I've been attending Calvary Chapel, Fort Lauderdale, since I was eighteen years old. Pastor Bob Coy is not only my pastor, he's a treasured friend. For as long as I can remember, just before he signs his name, he writes: "Until the Whole World Hears."

I've always loved this. When I think about Bob's calling and ministry, it sums up his heart perfectly. A few years ago I decided it was time for me to come up with my own sign-off slogan. For a while it was "Ditching the Diet," then "Much Love." Eventually, however, I began to realize neither of these offered serious hope. So I came up with something new, and I've stuck with it ever since: "Staying the Course, Chantel."

"Staying the Course" is my life's mantra for lots of reasons. Because of my own weight loss journey and ongoing wellness campaign, I am on a mission to remain on track. However, above all else I want to stay the course God has designed for every area of my life. I want to remain in the center of His will. I want to walk so close to Him I can feel His breath.

Walking with God is something that should consume us. When we decide to walk with Him, we are choosing to allow God to be our navigation system.

Six months ago, I entered the world of Apple by purchasing an iPhone. I'm no genius, but the whole company seems like a parallel universe. Now that I own this phone, I seem to have joined an elite group, as if I'm now a member of some secret society of the computer savvy. In reality, several billing cycles later, I feel that I'm just stupid enough to have allowed myself to be forced into buying products that have an exclusive "i" in front of them.

One of the features I have is texting. I am actually becoming pretty good at it. However, I'm starting to wonder if it's one of those technological advancements we are told to love, but should really hate. I'll admit it—I've been involved in a few misunderstandings due to this so-called communications breakthrough. As far as I'm concerned, texting is just an instant telegraph with an increased element of danger. Think about it. The beauty of taking the time to come up with a thoughtful response is gone. Plus, texting deprives you of the ability to hear the inflection of the other person's words. I asked my eleven-year-old son why he never calls his friends, and instead only texts them. His response, "Mom, calling someone is something you don't do until you're at least thirty!"

So I'm officially old, I guess, because I'd much rather hear someone speak back to me than have a screen-to-screen chat. If anything, I think texting may take us back in time. Now, instead of hearing the wonder of a live voice on the other end of the line, we must dissect a new language of shorthand in order to understand what the other person is trying to say. "TTYL" and "LOL" are just a few "text" catchphrases. Then there is the question of putting a smiley face at the end of a statement: do you put the colon ":)" or semi-colon ";)"? One is a nice smile, the other implies a wink. And what are you winking for? Is it just to be super friendly, or because you want to trade the inside scoop? It's too exhausting to be hip!

I've found out staying any course, including that of technology, requires some tricks. When it comes to the world of computers and text messaging, I will be on top of it for awhile. I'll text everyone, update my Facebook regularly, and so on. Then I'll wake up and decide to scrap the whole thing for a day or so. I will exclusively phone people and I'll refuse to leave a "detailed message" in their voice mail. Instead I just keep calling them back until they answer (like in the old days), and I treat checking my email like it's the post office on a holiday: it's unavailable. I apologize if you don't like what I'm saying; however, I want to help you. Sometimes we just need a break.

The only way to stay the course is to take scheduled breaks, recognize roadblocks—and then sometimes eat, breathe, and sleep success.

To Stay the Course, Take a Break

Every football fan has heard the term "bye week." Andy Cohen, a writer for the Miami Dolphins, says "The bye week gives you a chance to both reflect and look ahead."[10] A bye week is basically a scheduled break from competition. During this time, a team is able to practice fundamentals, nurse injuries, and prepare for the next game.

Taking a break from your regular wellness routine is essential. It gives your body time to recuperate. And it gives your mind time to refocus on your primary goals without the added pressure of "having" to do something.

Many people quit doing something they are succeeding at, simply because they lose their passion for the cause due to the pressure to maintain momentum. Someone who joins the gym the first week in January and goes faithfully for a month straight will often end up quitting entirely. Why? Usually it's because they begin to equate becoming a disciplined person with being someone who never takes a break. Therefore, when their body begins to become exhausted and their mind feels drained of focus, a sense of failure takes over and they give up.

If this has been you, it's okay—because it's been me, too! I've experienced the frustration of trying to stay on many courses, and I've learned the beauty of giving myself a "bye" from my regular routine.

A bye is a scheduled break. It isn't time off due to poor planning or lack of motivation. In other words, you don't say to yourself one morning, when the weather shows a 20 percent chance of rain, that it's the perfect time to skip your walk!

Most coaches report feeling itchy during a bye week, especially if they are on a winning streak. They often fear the team will relax too much. The only effective approach to taking a rest period is to know in advance when it's coming and to have a loose itinerary for the extra time.

I've designed the Walk with Him program to be five days a week. However, with the need to include strength training and focus on healthy eating, it's easy to feel like you're never getting a break. Don't get caught in a trap and wind up ensnared by your initial success. In other words, take one day off a week—and do nothing. Don't exercise, don't count calories, don't answer the phone (if you don't feel like it), and don't waste energy on anyone or anything that doesn't encourage or inspire you.

Now, I know this is a tall order. In fact, this may be extremely tough for some of you. "But Chantel, what do I do if it's my spouse or my child that seems to always suck the life out of me?" you may ask. To this I say: while you may not be able to take a physical break, take an emotional one. For this one day, forget they drive you crazy. Don't respond to negativity in your life. Take a break from your worries. Use the time off to pray, read, listen to your favorite music, or bake your famous chocolate chip cookies.

Roadblocks Are Real Life

If you want to stay the course, you'll need to know what to do in the event of a roadblock. I have taken many road trips that include some sort of roadblock along the way. When this happens, it can be pretty annoying. No one wants to be forced to take a different route, especially if we think it's going to make us late, or it seems out of the way. But what if the roadblock is due to new construction that will widen the road for the next time you need it? Would you see the detour in a different light? Of course you would. And what if the roadblock also gave you an extra hour to spend chatting with your daughter just before dropping her off at college? This may turn the unwelcome diversion into a meaningful conversation you will never forget.

As we approach a roadblock, choices will always present themselves. We can decide to turn around and go back or pull off to the side, take the key out of the ignition, and cry—or we can take the detour and continue in the direction we set out on, knowing we'll eventually get to our destination.

I'm honest enough to tell you that in the past I've been guilty of doing all three. However, I want to see you stay on track alongside me from now on. Over the past ten years, I've seen my course take many different routes. And I am still as committed to the destination as I was when I set out to reach it. What is your destination?

Since the night I began this journey, my destination has remained the same: "To be the best I can be." Some days I just hit cruise control and life seems to sail along; other days I am involved in a fender-bender, and I must assess the damage and have some repairs done. I imagine there are those of you who have been in a few head-on collisions, and you are nervous about getting behind the wheel ever again, let alone trying to stay on any course. Your life has been full of major events that make you constantly feel like you're in a tailspin. Here's hope: staying the course is something you don't need to do alone. God wants to be alongside you each and every day.

Eat, Breathe, and Sleep . . . Success

I remember when, back in college, I needed to get a passing grade in biology or I would be forced to retake the class the following semester. I had no choice. I had to eat, breathe, and sleep biology for several days.

I am far from being a science person. My all-time favorite courses in college were public speaking, world religion, and English literature. Biology was torture. But I knew the risks of avoiding it, and I wasn't willing to take them. So with lots of caffeine and little sleep, I became a temporary biology geek. You name it—I knew it. And I did pass the class with flying colors.

I can guarantee there will be times you need to eat, breathe, and sleep the feeling of success. Especially if you have been in a slight slump or are feeling unmotivated. The only way to get over a hump is to have power and speed. If you have ever pedaled a bike uphill, you know exactly what I'm talking about.

Getting speed and gaining power can come only from intense focus. I know it sounds like I'm telling you that staying the course requires first taking a break and then becoming slightly obsessive, but this isn't what I'm saying at all. If you are lacking drive, clear out some time in your schedule and double your efforts. This may mean you should go for a long walk in the morning and another one at night. It may be that you should stop eating sugar for a week and concentrate on eating more raw vegetables. Regardless of how you choose to get there, you need on occasion to feel the wind at your back. You won't appreciate how amazing that feels unless you have forced yourself to ride against it for awhile.

Begin to see your life's journey of healthy living as a child you have given birth to. Some days you'll need to give it special attention, some days you'll need to back off a bit, and some days you'll need to see the good and look past the bad. No matter what, your connection and commitment to staying the course will be with you for the rest of your life.

Epilogue

Welcome to the Tour de Life

*I*f you have never heard of the Tour de France, check it out. Don't let the name fool you. It may sound like a sweet little bicycle ride over some hillsides in Europe. Along the way, you'd likely imagine stopping for a warm croissant, or taking a break from pedaling to taste some delicious cheese. But before you cash in your retirement and book the trip, you should know the Tour de France is the furthest thing from all of that.

The Tour de France is actually a bike race that began in 1906. It takes place each year in the summer. Not only does it cover several thousand miles in a three-week span, it also includes riding at high elevations. After becoming a spinning instructor and purchasing a road bike, I became quite fascinated with the sport of cycling, and I'd look forward to this event each year. I can remember often getting up in the middle of the night throughout the month of July so I could catch some of the race live on television.

I had heard many experts and commentators describe the Tour de France as the most grueling athletic event of all time. Some have described it as running one marathon after another for several days in a row while making it to the top of Mount Everest approximately three times. The only reason I can figure why anyone would want to attempt this is maybe the same reason I found myself training for a marathon: I wanted to push my mental and physical limits to a height most people would only dream of reaching.

Every great achievement comes with great sacrifice. And the greater the accomplishment, the greater the cost to attain it will be. This is really the only way it can be considered "great" in the first place. Do I think these sacrifices are usually worth it?

Honestly, sometimes yes and sometimes no. Every finish line experience I've had has been amazing. I could never put a price tag on them. Even with all the pain along the way, the loss of a few toenails, and some minor dehydration, I still finished with a great feeling I could share with those I love. But I also can't put a price on the day-to-day enjoyment I have as a wife, mom, and writer. If I had to choose one or the other, my ordinary life or my extraordinary medals, I wouldn't need more than a moment to decide.

I read Lance Armstrong's first book, *It's Not About the Bike*. Most people know him as a seven-time winner of the Tour de France. I would have needed to be half-dead to miss the inspiring true story of a man who faced three forms of cancer, only to rebound and win the most prestigious cycling race many times over.

But as I finished this autobiography, I just wanted to cry. I had trouble celebrating the human spirit and Lance's success for more than the time it took to shut the book. Lance boldly called himself an agnostic, saying,

At the end of the day, if there was indeed some body or presence standing there to judge me, I hoped I would be judged on whether I had lived a true life, not on whether I believed in a certain book, or whether I'd been baptized. If there was indeed a god at the end of my days, I hoped he didn't say, "But you were never a Christian, so you're going the other way from heaven." If so, I was going to reply, "You know what? You're right. Fine."[11]

Here a man recovers from cancer, yet has no belief system in place to give the glory or credit to his Creator for a body strong enough to endure this disease. Lance also can't recognize there is a Creator who formed the minds of the doctors who discovered the drugs used to help treat him. And he also doesn't know the God who made the hands used to perform lifesaving surgery on him.

In God's mercy, He allowed Lance to live, and yet Lance is clueless, with only some really special video footage of a few memorable moments on a podium accepting his "wins." And the world will have trouble seeing what he's lost in the meantime.

Since Lance wanted more than anything to be a champion, he sacrificed being close to home and was away from his wife and children for months at a time. Eventually he disconnected from them, and filed for divorce. Just imagine what kind of message this sends to his kids, when one day they have a boss who insinuates they should skip their own child's first football game to entertain clients.

I don't share this to be critical of Lance or to imply his heart couldn't have shifted since the book was written; however, I am troubled when we elevate any human for success that has such a huge price tag attached to it. It's a dangerous thing and a very slippery slope. While Lance won the Tour de France, he may have lost the Tour de Life.

So far, my own Tour de Life has been full of surprises. Because of my longtime weight struggles, writing motivational books about fitness was something I could never have planned to do. In fact, to this day, when I'm asked "What do you do?" and I respond, "I write books," I begin to feel a nervous twitch as twenty more questions follow.

In the past, this conversation possessed the power to send me swimming in a sea of self-doubt. And trying to answer all those questions well made me feel like I'd never make it to shore. I've begun to accept that tumultuous waters are part of any great journey. But at the same time, we all must consider the cost of every passion we pursue. This is the only hope we have in winning the only race that has an eternal prize.

The Tour de Life is about making regular choices to do things that will help you leave a legacy of everlasting hope for those you love, just like my Pepa did. When we walk with God, He will always keep us on course to win the Tour de Life, pursuing the things that matter most. While many of these things may occasionally seem boring or repetitive, the payoff God guarantees is indescribable.

When it comes to encouraging others along the way, remember that recalling some details of your past can be helpful, which is why I've shared some of mine with you. However, the overall message I pray you'll always hear from me is this: I am simply a woman who finally found that looking up is the only way I can walk strong and remain at the front of the pack in the Tour de Life. An accumulation of hours, days, weeks, months, and miles spent "walking" physically, emotionally, and spiritually with Him has given me ultimate hope for the win: an eternal home in heaven celebrating 24/7 with my Savior!

Before you close this book, please make sure you're on the right Tour. We can share the prize. There is absolutely no cap on the number of victors in the Tour de Life. God desires for all of His children to make it over this finish line. In fact, it's only through the cross we are able to "cross" it! Please don't make the giant mistake of squandering time on a "tour de depression and frustration" when the ultimate Tour de Everlasting Life is waiting for you today!

Notes

1. C. S. Lewis, *Mere Christianity* (New York: Harper One, 1952), 135.

2. "The Worry Tree!" Piffe the Puffin, accessed March 29, 2011, http://www.naute.com/stories/worrytree.phtml.

3. "Record Heat in South Florida," *The Fort Lauderdale News and Real Estate Report*, posted September 30, 2010, http://www.robinashley.com/tag/record-heat-in-south-florida/.

4. "Assessing Your Weight and Health Risk," National Heart, Lung, and Blood Institute, accessed February 22, 2011, http://www.nhlbi.nih.gov/health/public/heart/obesity/lose_wt/risk.htm.

5. Statistics here are taken from Elisa Zeid, *Nutrition at Your Fingertips* (New York: Alpha, 2009).

6. http://www.iom.edu.

7. "NWCR Facts," The National Weight Control Registry, accessed March 29, 2011, http://www.nwcr.ws/Research/default.htm.

8. "Strength Training," The Free Dictionary, accessed March 1, 2011, http://medical-dictionary.thefreedictionary.com/Strength+training.

9. Paul Johnson, *Jesus* (Waterville, ME: Thorndike Press, 2010), 396.

10. Andy Cohen, "Andy Cohen's Bye Week Reflections: Dolphins Still a Good Team," posted October 12, 2010, http://www.miamidolphins.com/news/andy-cohens-bye-week-reflection-dolphins-still-good-team.

11. Lance Armstrong and Sally Jenkins, *It's Not About the Bike: My Journey Back to Life* (New York: Berkley Books, 2001), 113.

Chantel Hobbs is a life coach, personal trainer, marathon runner, wife, and mother of four. Her amazing story of losing two hundred pounds and keeping the weight off has been featured on *Oprah*, *The Today Show*, *Good Morning America*, *Fox & Friends*, *Life Today with James Robison*, *The 700 Club*, *Focus on the Family Radio*, and in *People* and *First* magazines. Chantel is a featured fitness expert on nationally syndicated radio programs. She is also a frequent speaker to women's groups and makes personal appearances at fitness conventions.

The developer of the One-Day Way Learning System and the author of several books including *Never Say Diet* and *The One-Day Way*, Chantel lives with her family in South Florida. Visit her at www.faithfoodandfitness.com for advice, fitness updates, coaching tips, and answers to your healthy-living questions.